RESPIRATORY THERAPY

EXAMINATION REVIEW

600 **MULTIPLE-CHOICE QUESTIONS WITH EXPLANATORY ANSWERS**

Galen G. Heath, RRT
Manager, Respiratory Services

John M. Gallagher, RRT
Quality Assurance/Educational Coordinator
Respiratory Services

The Mercy Hospital of Pittsburgh
Pittsburgh, Pennsylvania

Respiratory Therapist Advisory Board
Wheeling Jesuit College
Wheeling, West Virginia
and
Jefferson Technical College
Steubenville, Ohio

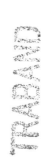

MEDICAL EXAMINATION PUBLISHING COMPANY

Medical Examination Publishing Company
A Division of Elsevier Science Publishing Co., Inc.
655 Avenue of the Americas, New York, New York 10010

© 1991 by Elsevier Science Publishing Co., Inc.

This book has been registered with the Copyright Clearance Center, Inc. For further information, please contact the Copyright Clearance Center, Inc., Salem, Massachusetts.

Library of Congress Cataloging-in-Publication Data

Heath, Galen.
    Respiratory therapy examination review : 600 multiple-choice questions with explanatory answers / Galen Heath, John Gallagher.
        p.   cm.
    Includes bibliographical references.
    ISBN 0-444-01571-X (alk. paper)
    1. Respiratory therapy—Examinations, questions, etc.
I. Gallagher, John, 1961–   II. Title.
    [DNLM: 1. Respiratory Therapy—examination questions.   WB 18
H437r]
RM161.H45   1990
616.2′0046—dc20
DNLM/DLC
for Library of Congress   90-13638
                                                                        CIP

Current printing (last digit):
10 9 8 7 6 5 4 3 2 1

Manufactured in the United States of America

*To our families for their support and understanding
and to Sharon for her patience.*

Contents

vi / Contents

Preface

Respiratory Therapy Examination Review was written primarily for students preparing to take the entry level certifying examination administered by the National Board for Respiratory Care (NBRC). It is designed to give you an opportunity to improve your knowledge of respiratory procedures, equipment, and practice while providing experience with the written testing process used by the NBRC.

Through the use of multiple-choice questions in the same format as that used by the NBRC, you will be able to identify areas of strength and weakness in your own command of the subjects presented. Detailed explanatory answers, referenced to a variety of information sources, follow each section of questions. This useful feature allows you to return to the authoritative reference for further study.

Respiratory Therapy Examination Review will help you organize your valuable study time and use it more efficiently. You will also become familiar with the style and format of the certifying exam, thus gaining a psychological edge as well.

1 Gases and Gas Laws

DIRECTIONS (Questions 1–23): Each of the questions or incomplete statements below is followed by four suggested answers or completions. Select the **one** that is **best** in each case.

1. Atmospheric pressure at sea level is
   1. 760 mmHg
   2. 14.7 lb/in.²
   3. 29.9 in. Hg
   4. 47 mmHg
      A. 1. and 2.
      B. 1., 2., and 3.
      C. 1. only
      D. 4. only

2. The atmosphere is composed of what percentage of oxygen?
   A. 78.09%
   B. 20.94%
   C. 25.04%
   D. 16.40%

3. The atmosphere is composed of what percentage of nitrogen?
   A. 78.09%
   B. 20.94%
   C. 0.93%
   D. 0.04%

4. Carbon dioxide composes what percentage of the atmosphere?
   A. 20.94%
   B. 0.93%
   C. 0.04%
   D. 3.00%

5. The absolute humidity of respiratory gases at 37°C is
   A. 37 mmHg
   B. 45 mmHg
   C. 47 mmHg
   D. 50 mmHg

6. At a constant temperature the volume of gas is inversely proportional to the pressure. This is known as
   A. Charles' Law
   B. Boyle's Law
   C. Dalton's Law
   D. Henry's Law

7. At a constant pressure the volume of gas is directly proportional to the absolute temperature. This is known as
   A. Charles' Law
   B. Boyle's Law
   C. Henry's Law
   D. Dalton's Law

8. A mass of oxygen occupies a volume of 2 L at a pressure of 600 mmHg. To what pressure must the gas be subjected in order to change the volume to 750 mL (temperature is constant)?
   A. 2500 mmHg
   B. 2200 mmHg
   C. 1600 mmHg
   D. 2000 mmHg

9. 20°C is equal to (degrees Kelvin)
   A. 253K
   B. 293K
   C. 68K
   D. 43K

10. If a volume of gas occupies 5 L at 20°C, what is the new volume if the temperature is increased to 40°C and pressure is constant?
    A. 2.5 L
    B. 4.68 L
    C. 5.34 L
    D. 10 L

11. The law that states that in a mixture of gases, each exerts a pressure independent of the other gases present and that the total pressure is the arithmetical sum of the partial pressures exerted by each gas is
    A. Dalton's Law
    B. Charles' Law
    C. Avogadro's Law
    D. Boyle's Law

12. The critical temperature of a gas is the temperature
    A. at which a gas boils
    B. below which a gas cannot be liquefied
    C. above which a gas cannot exist as a liquid regardless of the amount of pressure applied.
    D. both A. and B.

13. The partial pressure of oxygen at sea level is
    A. 20 mmHg
    B. 100 mmHg
    C. 120 mmHg
    D. 159 mmHg

14. If the atmospheric pressure at 19,000 feet above sea level is 344 mmHg, the concentration of oxygen would be, approximately
    A. 21%
    B. 15%
    C. 10%
    D. 5%

15. One cubic foot of liquid oxygen equals how many cubic feet of gaseous oxygen?
    A. 760
    B. 400
    C. 860
    D. 2400

16. One cubic foot of gaseous oxygen equals how many liters of gaseous oxygen?
    A. 20.94
    B. 16
    C. 45
    D. 28.3

17. When a gas is compressed
    A. the space between the gas molecules decreases
    B. heat is given off
    C. there is an increase in pressure
    D. all of the above

18. All gases exert pressure when
    A. enclosed in a container
    B. dissolved in a liquid
    C. heated
    D. all of the above

19. Volumes of gases as they exist in the lungs are recorded as
    A. BTPS
    B. STPD
    C. ATPS
    D. none of the above

20. The abbreviation STPD means
   1. a volume of dry gas, at a temperature of 0°C and a PB of 760 mmHg
   2. a volume of dry gas, at a temperature of 37°C and a PB of 760 mmHg
   3. standard temperature and pressure, dry gas
   4. a volume of gas saturated with water vapor, at a temperature 0°C and PB of 760 mmHg
   A. 1. and 3.
   B. 2. only
   C. 1. only
   D. 2. and 3.

21. ATPS means
   A. a volume of dry gas at a temperature of 0°C and ambient pressure
   B. a volume of dry gas at a pressure of 760 mmHg and ambient temperature
   C. a volume of gas saturated with water vapor at ambient temperature and pressure
   D. none of the above

22. BTPS means
   A. a volume of gas saturated with water vapor, at 37°C and the ambient PB.
   B. a volume of dry gas at 37°C and the ambient PB.
   C. a volume of gas saturated with water vapor, at 0°C and ambient PB.
   D. a volume of dry gas at 0°C and a PB of 760 mmHg.

23. Given 100 mL of dry gas measured at 37°C and 760 mmHg, PB, what would its volume be at 800 mmHg?
   A. 95 mL
   B. 97 mL
   C. 102 mL
   D. 107 mL

Explanatory Answers

1. B. There are several methods of expressing normal atmospheric pressure at sea level. Among these are 760 mmHg, 14.7 lb/in.^{2}, and 29.9 in. Hg. 47 mmHg represents the partial pressure of water vapor at 37°C. (**Ref.** 6, p. 21)

2. B. Oxygen exerts a partial pressure of 20.94% of the total atmospheric pressure. This corresponds to a Po_2 of 149. (760 mmHg − 47 mmHg .2094) at 37°C, sea level. (**Ref.** 6, p. 22)

3. A. Nitrogen comprises 78.09% of the total atmospheric pressure or a partial pressure of the total atmospheric pressure of 557 mmHg at 37°C and sea level (760 mmHg − 47 mmHg .7809). (**Ref.** 6, p. 22)

4. C. Carbon dioxide comprises .04% of the total atmospheric pressure or a partial pressure of the total atmospheric pressure of .29 mmHg at 37°C and at sea level. (**Ref.** 6, p. 22)

5. C. The absolute humidity of respiratory gases at 37°C or the partial pressure of water vapor is expressed at $P_{H_2O} = 47$ mmHg. Water vapor is the only standard atmospheric gas that changes its concentration with changes in temperature. As temperature increases the capacity for atmosphere to hold water increases. (**Ref.** 6, p. 22)

6. B. Boyle's Law states that if temperature is constant, volume and pressure are inversely proportional, such that when pressure on a gas is doubled, volume will be reduced by one-half. Boyle's Law is written $P_1V_1 = P_2V_2$. (**Ref.** 6, p. 22)

7. A. Charles' Law states that if pressure remains constant, volume is directly proportional to the change in absolute temperature (Kelvin). If pressure is constant and temperature is doubled, volume is doubled. Charles' Law is written as $\dfrac{V_1}{V_2} = \dfrac{T_1}{T_2}$ (**Ref.** 6, p. 22)

8. C. By utilizing Boyle's Law: $P_1V_1 = P_1V_2$ we can solve for X or the unknown pressure.

1. $P_1 \times V_2$ (750 mL) = P_2 (600 mmHg) V_2 (2000 mL)

2. $P_1 = \dfrac{600 \text{ mmHg} \times 2000 \text{ mL}}{750 \text{ mL}}$

3. $P_1 = 1,200,000/750 = 1600$ mmHg (**Ref.** 6, p. 23)

9. B. Kelvin can be calculated by adding degrees centigrade to 273. This scale was developed to account for absolute (perfect) zero. Zero degrees Kelvin represents the point where all molecular activity stops. Therefore, $20°C$ is equivalent to $20° + 273°$ or 293K. (**Ref.** 6, p. 23)

10. C. Since pressure is constant, the new volume can be solved for by utilizing Charles' Law $\dfrac{V_1}{V_2} = \dfrac{T_1}{T_2}$ The first step is to convert temperature to Kelvin

$\dfrac{V_1}{V_2}$ (5 L) = $\dfrac{(20°C + 273) \text{ T1}}{(40°C + 273) \text{ T2}}$

$\dfrac{5}{V_2} = .936$

$5 \text{ L} = .936 \times V2$

$\dfrac{5 \text{ L}}{.936} = V_2$

$5.34 = V_2$ (**Ref.** 6, p. 23)

11. A. Dalton's Law states that in a mixture of gases, each gas will exert a partial pressure independent of one another and that the total pressure is the sum of the partial pressures of each gas. Avogadro's Theory states that one mole of any ideal gas has an equal number of molecules of another gas of identical volume independent of temperature or pressure. (**Ref.** 6, p. 24)

12. C. The critical temperature is the highest temperature at which gases can remain at their liquid state regardless of the amount of pressure applied to it. (**Ref.** 7, p. 12)

13. D. The partial pressure of oxygen at sea level (760 mmHg) is equivalent to 760 mmHg $\times$ .2094 (partial pressure of oxygen) = P_{O_2} of 159 mmHg. (**Ref.** 7, p. 12)

14. A. Regardless of atmospheric pressure, so long as you remain within the earth's atmosphere, the concentration of oxygen will always be 21%. (**Ref.** 7, p. 12)

15. C. At its boiling point, 1 ft^3 of liquid oxygen is equivalent to 860 ft^3 of gaseous oxygen at ambient temperature and pressure. (**Ref.** 7, p. 278)

16. D. Gas may be converted from cubic feet into liters by 1 ft^3 = 28.316 L. (**Ref.** 7, p. 273)

17. D. According to Gay–Lussac's Law, if volume is constant and pressure increases by compressing the gas, temperature is directly proportional to pressure. The gas molecules occupy a smaller area causing an increase in pressure. Therefore, the answer is all of the above.

18. D. All gases exert pressure whether free in atmosphere or enclosed in a container heated or cooled. Gases dissolved in liquid also will exert pressure. This is referred to as the tension of a gas. (**Ref.** 7, p. 2)

19. A. Volumes of gases are recorded as BTPS as they exist in the lungs. This means saturated with water vapor at 37°C (body temperature) at ambient barometric pressure STPD refers to a dry gas and ATPS refers to a gas at room temperature. (**Ref.** 7, p. 16)

20. A. STPD refers to a volume of dry gas at a temperature of 0°C and a barometric pressure of 760 mmHg. The abbreviation stands for standard temperature and pressure deviation. (**Ref.** 7, p. 16)

21. A. ATPS refers to ambient temperature and pressure saturated. It is a volume of gas saturated at room temperature and ambient barometric pressure. (**Ref.** 7, p. 16)

22. A. BTPS refers to body temperature and pressure saturated. It is a volume of gas saturated at $37°C$ and at ambient barometric pressure. (**Ref.** 7, p. 16)

23. A. By utilizing at combined gas law

$$V_2 = \frac{V_1 \times P_1 \times T_2}{P_2 \times T_1}$$

Temperature must be converted from celsius to Kelvin $37°C + 273 = 310°$

The new pressure would be $= \dfrac{100 \text{ mL} \times 760 \times 310}{800 \times 310}$

$V_2 = 95$ mL (**Ref.** 7, p. 23)

2 Pulmonary Physiology

DIRECTIONS (Questions 24–33): Each of the questions or incomplete statements below is followed by four suggested answers or completions. Select the **one** that is **best** in each case.

24. The objectives of breathing exercises are
    1. promoting a normal relaxed pattern of breathing, where possible
    2. teaching controlled breathing with the minimum amount of effort
    3. assisting with removal of secretions
    4. aiding re-expansion of lung tissue
    5. mobilizing the thoracic cage
        A. 1., 2., and 3.
        B. 1., 3., and 5.
        C. 1., 2., 3., and 4.
        D. all of the above

25. Diaphragmatic breathing, if performed properly, can be used
    A. during attacks of dyspnea
    B. to improve ventilation
    C. to loosen secretions in the base of the lungs
    D. all of the above

10

26. When instructing the patient to perform diaphragmatic breathing
    A. the patient should be positioned so that his/her back and head are fully supported and abdominal wall relaxed
    B. a high-back chair without arms is most suitable
    C. the therapist's hands should rest lightly on the anterior costal margins to stimulate and palpate the movement occurring
    D. all of the above

27. Which of the following are common faults of diaphragmatic breathing?
    1. Forced expiration
    2. Prolonged expiration
    3. Overuse of upper chest and accessory muscles
       A. 2. and 3.
       B. 1. and 2.
       C. 1. only
    4. All of the above

28. Which of the following localized expansion exercises is indicated for apical pneumothorax?
    1. Upper lateral expansion
    2. Apical expansion
    3. Unilateral basal expansion
    4. Bilateral basal expansion
       A. 1. and 2.
       B. 2. only
       C. 4. only
       D. None of the above

29. When performing postural drainage
   1. the patient is positioned to assist the drainage of secretions from specific areas of the lungs by gravity
   2. it is advisable to carry out postural drainage immediately after a meal
   3. vibratory shaking or percussion of chest should be performed
   4. it should be performed immediately before meals
   - **A.** 1. and 3.
   - **B.** 1., 3., and 4.
   - **C.** 1. only
   - **D.** all of the above

30. The proper position for postural drainage of the right posterior bronchus is
   - **A.** lying on right side turned 45 deg. onto face, with shoulders lifted 12 in. from bed
   - **B.** lying on left side turned 45 deg. onto face, with shoulders lifted 12 in. from bed
   - **C.** lying flat on face, pillow under hips
   - **D.** lying on right side with a pillow under hips, foot of bed raised 18 in.

31. Having the patient lying flat on his/her back, body quarter turned to right, maintained by a pillow under left side from shoulder to hip, foot of bed raised 14 in., is used to drain
   - **A.** lingula lobe
   - **B.** lower lobe
   - **C.** middle lobe
   - **D.** upper lobe

32. Diaphragmatic breathing is
   - **A.** breathing with diaphragm only
   - **B.** breathing controlled by correct use of the diaphragm
   - **C.** using abdominal muscles primarily to push the diaphragm upward
   - **D.** forced inspiration by draining the abdominal muscles inward

33. Which of the following is incorrect?
   A. A patient should take a deep breaths before coughing
   B. The abdominal muscles should relax during cough
   C. If a patient persists in coughing without breathing in, syncope occurs
   D. The patient should contract his/her abdominal muscles during cough

14 / Respiratory Therapy Examination Review

Explanatory Answers

24. D. Promoting a relaxed pattern of breathing with a minimal amount of effort, along with assisting in the removal of secretions, re-expansion of lung tissue, and mobilization of the thoracic cage are all objectives of breathing exercises. (**Ref.** 8, p. 5)

25. D. Diaphragmatic breathing is done by palpating the patient for anterior costal motion to improve ventilation, loosen secretions in the bases, and alleviate attacks of dyspnea. (**Ref.** 8, p. 6)

26. D. Patient should be comfortably positioned with full back support, with the therapist's hands palpating the anterior costal margins to stimulate diaphragmatic movement. (**Ref.** 8, p. 5)

27. D. In diaphragmatic breathing, expiration should be passive without encouragement for complete exhalation. Accessory muscle use should be discouraged as it leads to inefficient diaphragm use and increased oxygen demand. (**Ref.** 8, p. 6)

28. B. Apical pneumothoracies can be helped by apical expansion. This is accomplished by expanding the chest against pressure applied by the fingers just below the clavicle. (**Ref.** 8, p. 8)

29. A. Postural drainage is the process of utilizing gravity to drain secretions from specific areas of the lung. It should not be done follwing meals so as not to induce aspiration. Vibratory shaking is a separate modality used in conjunction with postural drainage to eliminate secretions. (**Ref.** 8, p. 11)

30. B. The posterior bronchus of the right upper lobe is drained by lying on the left side turned 45 deg. onto the face, with the shoulders lifted 12 in. from the bed. (**Ref.** 8, p. 13)

31. A. The superior and inferior bronchus of the lingular lobe is drained by having the patient lie flat on his/her back turned a quarter to the right with a pillow under the left side. The foot of the bed is elevated 14 in. (**Ref.** 8, p. 13)

32. B. Diaphragmatic breathing is best described as breathing controlled by correct use of the diaphragm. It is done in a relaxed fashion with discouragement of forced inspiration or exhalation. (**Ref.** 8, p. 5)

33. B. Coughing should be preceded by deep breaths and contractions of the abdominal muscles to aid in the buildup of pressure. If uncontrolled coughing persists, syncope can occur. Diaphagmatic breathing should be interspersed between bouts of coughing. (**Ref.** 8, pp. 10, 11)

3 Cardiopulmonary Anatomy and Physiology

DIRECTIONS (Questions 34–131): Each of the questions or incomplete statements below is followed by four suggested answers or completions. Select the **one** that is **best** in each case.

34. The nasal cavities perform the following functions
    A. filter inspired air
    B. transport particulate matter toward the external nares discharge
    C. humidify and warm inspired air
    D. all of the above

35. The pharynx is divided into which of the following regions?
    1. Larynx
    2. Nasopharynx
    3. Laryngopharynx
    4. Oropharynx
       A. 2. and 3.
       B. 2., 3., and 4.
       C. 1. and 3.
       D. All of the above

36. The trachea in the average adult is, approximately, how long?
    1. 12 cm
    2. 16 cm
    3. 4.5 to 5.5 in.
    4. 8.5 to 9.5 in.
        A. 1. only
        B. 2. and 3.
        C. 1. and 3.
        D. 4. only

37. The diameter of the trachea in the average adult is
    A. 0.5 to 1.5 cm
    B. 1.5 to 2.5 cm
    C. 2.0 to 3.0 cm
    D. 2.5 to 3.5 cm

38. The trachea contains how many C-shaped cartilaginous rings?
    A. 12 to 14
    B. 16 to 20
    C. 18 to 22
    D. 20 to 24

39. Anatomically, the trachea begins and ends at which two sites?
    A. Laryngopharynx and its subdivision
    B. Larynx and bronchiole
    C. Larynx and its subdivision
    D. Laryngopharynx and bronchiole

40. The primary muscle of respiration, whose main function is to initiate inspiration, is
    A. the diaphragm
    B. the abdominal
    C. the intercostal
    D. accessory muscles

41. Each lung is surrounded by the pleural surface which consists of two layers. The layer closely applied to the lung is called
    A. parietal pleura
    B. pneumo pleura
    C. visceral pleura
    D. thorax pleura

42. The layer of the pleural surface applied to the chest wall is called
    A. parietal pleura
    B. pneumo pleura
    C. visceral pleura
    D. thorax pleura

43. Each lung is divided into lobes. The left lung contains how many lobes?
    A. 2
    B. 3
    C. 4
    D. 5

44. The right lung consists of which of the following lobes?
    1. Upper lobe
    2. Middle lobe
    3. Lower lobe
    4. Frontal lobe
        A. 1. and 3.
        B. 1., 2., and 3.
        C. 2. and 3.
        D. All of the above

45. The anatomical deadspace consists of which of the following?
   1. Nose
   2. Pharynx
   3. Trachea
   4. Bronchi
   5. Terminal bronchioles
      A. 1., 2., and 3.
      B. 1. and 3.
      C. 1., 2., 3., and 4.
      D. All of the above

46. Both lungs contain, approximately, how many alveoli?
   A. 300,000
   B. 300,000,000
   C. 500,000
   D. 500,000,000

47. The number of generations of branches of the respiratory system is
   A. 16
   B. 18
   C. 23
   D. 27

48. The rib cage is composed of how many pairs of ribs?
   A. 7
   B. 10
   C. 12
   D. 14

49. How many pairs of ribs are attached to the sternum by the costal cartilage?
   A. 3
   B. 7
   C. 10
   D. 12

50. The exchange of oxygen for carbon dioxide in the alveolus is known as
    A. ventilation
    B. internal respiration
    C. external respiration
    D. none of the above

51. Rapid shallow breathing is defined as which of the following terms
    A. tachypnea
    B. polypnea
    C. hyperventilation
    D. orthopnea

52. Where breathing may be more comfortable in a particular position is described as
    A. trepopnea
    B. ponopnea
    C. polypnea
    D. orthopnea

53. Short rapid breathing episodes interrupted by 10 to 30 sec pauses is
    A. Cheyne – Stokes' ventilation
    B. Biot's ventilation
    C. Kussmaul's ventilation
    D. polypnea

54. Cyclic changes in breathing pattern: respiration stops for 5 to 30 sec and resumes with gradual increase in volume of breathing and then gradually decreases in intensity until another pause occurs. This describes
    A. apnea
    B. Boit's ventilation
    C. Cheyne – Stokes' ventilation
    D. oligopnea ventilation

55. Conscious realization (by patient) of the effort of breathing (distressed or laborious respiration) describes
    A. eupnea
    B. dyspnea
    C. hypoventilation
    D. apneustic ventilation

56. Presence of normal spontaneous breathing is described as
    A. orthopnea
    B. trepopnea
    C. eupnea
    D. ponopnea

57. Increased depth of breathing describes
    A. hyperventilation
    B. hyperpnea
    C. hypoventilation
    D. polypnea

58. Breathing at a rate and depth in excess of that required to maintain arterial P_{CO_2} and increased pH describes
    A. hypoventilation
    B. hyperpnea
    C. hyperventilation
    D. polypnea

59. Breathing at a rate and depth below that which is required to maintain arterial P_{CO_2} at 40 mmHg (results in an increased arterial P_{CO_2} and decreased pH) describes
    A. hypoventilation
    B. hyperpnea
    C. ponopnea
    D. trepopnea

60. Distressing shortness of breath (air hunger) occurring spasmodically and a warning of diabetic crisis describes
    A. Kussmaul's ventilation
    B. Boit's ventilation
    C. oligopnea
    D. trepopnea

61. The term used to describe slowed breathing or breathing of small volume is
   A. oligopnea
   B. orthopnea
   C. ponopnea
   D. tachypnea

62. The term used to describe inability to breathe except in upright position is
   A. orthopnea
   B. oligopnea
   C. ponopnea
   D. trepopnea

63. The term used to define rapid breathing is
   A. polypnea
   B. hyperventilation
   C. tachypnea
   D. oligopnea

64. Painful breathing is defined by which of the following terms?
   A. Ponopnea
   B. Trepopnea
   C. Orthopnea
   D. Apnea

65. The exchange of oxygen and carbon dioxide takes place between the blood and the atmospheric air at which areas?
   1. Terminal bronchioles
   2. Respiratory bronchioles
   3. Alveolar ducts
   4. Alveolar atria
      A. 1. and 2.
      B. 2., 3., and 4.
      C. 4. only
      D. All of the above

66. The exchange of oxygen for carbon dioxide between the blood and tissue cells is referred to as
    A. tissue ventilation
    B. internal respiration
    C. external respiration
    D. cellular respiration

67. A fully saturated cubic meter of air at 37°C can hold
    A. 48.9 grams of water
    B. 43.8 grams of water
    C. 52.5 grams of water
    D. 37.8 grams of water

68. The percentage of total blood volume which consists of erythrocytes is termed
    A. hematocyte
    B. hemolysis
    C. hematocrit
    D. hemoglobin

69. The normal hematocrit range for an adult female at sea level is
    A. 37% to 47%
    B. 40% to 54%
    C. 35% to 49%
    D. 49% to 54%

70. The normal hematocrit range for an adult male at sea level is
    A. 37% to 47%
    B. 40% to 54%
    C. 35% to 49%
    D. 49% to 54%

71. The iron-containing pigment of the red blood cells is
    A. hematocyte
    B. hemolysis
    C. hematocrit
    D. hemoglobin

72. The amount of hemoglobin in the blood for the adult male averages
    A. 14 to 18 g/100 mL of blood
    B. 12 to 16 g/100 mL of blood
    C. 10 to 14 g/100 mL of blood
    D. 16 to 20 g/100 mL of blood

73. The amount of hemoglobin in the blood for the adult female averages
    A. 14 to 18 g/100 mL of blood
    B. 12 to 16 g/100 mL of blood
    C. 10 to 14 g/100 mL of blood
    D. 16 to 20 g/100 mL of blood

74. The normal erythrocyte count in males is approximately
    A. 5,400,000 cells/mm^3 of blood
    B. 4,700,000 cells/mm^3 of blood
    C. 6,400,000 cells/mm^3 of blood
    D. 4,000,000 cells/mm^3 of blood

75. The normal erythrocyte count in females is approximately
    A. 5,400,000 cells/mm^3
    B. 4,700,000 cells/mm^3
    C. 6,400,000 cells/mm^3
    D. 4,000,000 cells/mm^3

76. Another name for red blood cells is
    A. macrophages
    B. thrombocytes
    C. leukocytes
    D. erythrocytes

77. Leukopenia is
    A. an increase in the number of white blood cells
    B. a reduction in the number of white blood cells
    C. the formation process of white blood cells
    D. another name for leukemia

78. Another name for white blood cells is
    A. macrophages
    B. thrombocytes
    C. leukocytes
    D. erythrocytes

79. The total leukocyte count ranges from
    A. 15,000 to 20,000
    B. 10,000 to 15,000
    C. 5,000 to 10,000
    D. 20,000 to 25,000

80. On a standard electrocardiogram, what wave shows the reflection of ventricular repolarization?
    A. R
    B. Q
    C. T
    D. P

81. When an abnormal ventricular beat is coupled to a normal sinus beat, this is referred to as
    A. ventricle bigeminy
    B. ventricular tachycardia
    C. premature ventricular contraction
    D. ventricular fibrillation

82. Myocardial conduction cells have characteristics closely resembling nervous tissue and are the cells which normally spread impulses. Which of these groups of cells are known as the pacemaker of the heart?
    A. SA node
    B. Perkinje's fibcrs
    C. AV node
    D. Bundle of His

83. What mechanism is involved in hemostasis?
    A. Platelet agulation
    B. Contraction of blood vessels
    C. Formation of a fibrin clot
    D. All of the above

84. What hemorrhagic disease is characterized by loss of blood into the skin, subcutaneous tissue, and mucus membrane?
  A. Thrombosis
  B. Purpura
  C. Hemophilia
  D. None of the above

85. In blood grouping, which type is the universal donor?
  A. O
  B. AB
  C. A
  D. None of the above

86. In blood grouping, which type is the universal recipient?
  A. AB
  B. B
  C. O
  D. A

87. The osmotic pressure of human blood is maintained by which of the following?
  A. Electrolytes
  B. Plasma protein
  C. Sugar
  D. All of the above

88. The walls of the heart consist of which of the following layers?
  A. Epicardium
  B. Myocardium
  C. Endocardium
  D. All of the above

89. The thickness of the myocardium varies. Which is the thickest section?
  A. Right atrium
  B. Right ventricle
  C. Left ventricle
  D. Left atrium

90. Which chamber of the heart does the vena cava empty into?
   A. Left atrium
   B. Left ventricle
   C. Right atrium
   D. Right ventricle

91. Which chamber of the heart sends blood to the lungs?
   A. Left ventricle
   B. Right atrium
   C. Left atrium
   D. Right ventricle

92. Which chamber of the heart sends blood through the aorta?
   A. Left ventricle
   B. Right atrium
   C. Left atrium
   D. Right ventricle

93. Which chamber of the heart receives blood from the lungs?
   A. Left ventricle
   B. Right atrium
   C. Left atrium
   D. Right ventricle

94. Which of the following valves are located between the atria and the ventricles?
   1. Pulmonary
   2. Mitral
   3. Aortic
   4. Tricuspid
      A. 3. and 4.
      B. 1., 2., and 4.
      C. 2. and 4.
      D. All of the above

95. The aortic valve guards the orifice between the aorta and
   A. right atrium
   B. left ventricle
   C. left atrium
   D. right ventricle

96. The pulmonary valve guards the orifice between the pulmonary arteries and
    A. left atrium
    B. right ventricle
    C. right atrium
    D. left ventricle

97. Irreversible damage to the brain can occur if cardiac massage is not started within how many minutes after the heart stops?
    A. 2 min
    B. 4 min
    C. 6 min
    D. 8 min

98. The wall of the heart consists of how many layers?
    A. 4
    B. 2
    C. 3
    D. None of the above

99. In the fetus the opening between the two atria is called
    A. ductus arteriosus
    B. foramen ovale
    C. ductus venosus
    D. none of the above

100. Which of the following is the blood vessel connecting the pulmonary artery with the aorta in a fetus?
    A. Foramen ovale
    B. Ductus venosus
    C. Ductus arteriosus
    D. None of the above

101. The initial stages of progressive shock are characterized by
  1. reduced BP
  2. shallow respirations
  3. rapid pulse
  4. cold skin
     A. 1. and 2.
     B. 1., 2., and 3.
     C. 1., 3., and 4.
     D. All of the above

102. The average volume of blood ejected by the heart per beat is
   A. 75 to 85 mL
   B. 40 to 50 mL
   C. 60 to 70 mL
   D. 45 to 55 mL

103. The inferior and superior venae cavae empty into what chamber of the heart?
   A. Right atrium
   B. Left atrium
   C. Right ventricle
   D. Left ventricle

104. What is the valve located between the left atrium and left ventricle?
   A. Pulmonary
   B. Mitral
   C. Tricuspid
   D. Aortic

105. What is the valve located between the right atrium and right ventricle?
   A. Pulmonary
   B. Mitral
   C. Tricuspid
   D. Aortic

106. Which heart block represents a total dissociation of the atrial and ventricular rhythms?
   A. First degree
   B. Second degree
   C. Third degree
   D. Fourth degree

107. When a prolonged PR interval is noted on the cardiogram which degree heart block is indicated?
   A. First
   B. Second
   C. Third
   D. Fourth

108. Which heart rhythm shows a cardiac rate of less than 60 beats/min?
   A. Sinus arrhythmia
   B. Sinus tachycardia
   C. Sinus bradycardia
   D. Normal sinus rhythm

109. Which heart rhythm shows a cardiac rate greater than 100 beats/min?
   A. Sinus arrhythmia
   B. Sinus tachycardia
   C. Sinus bradycardia
   D. Normal sinus rhythm

110. Which of the following components of the nerve fiber carries impulses to the cell body?
   A. Soma
   B. Dendrite
   C. Axon
   D. None of the above

111. Which of the following components of the nerve fiber carries impulses away from the cell body?
   A. Soma
   B. Dendrite
   C. Axon
   D. None of the above

112. Which neurons transmit nerve impulses to the brain?
   A. Sensory
   B. Motor
   C. Interneurons
   D. Soma

113. What is the junction between one neuron and another neuron, muscle, or gland?
   A. Nerve impulse
   B. Nerve synapse
   C. Nerve cell
   D. Neuromuscular junction

114. Which of the following decreases transmission across the synapse?
   A. Norepinephrine
   B. Alkalosis
   C. Acidosis
   D. Acetylcholine

115. Which of the following increases transmission across the synapse?
   A. Norepinephrine
   B. Alkalosis
   C. Acidosis
   D. Acetylcholine

116. Which of the following is a transmitter substance of the peripheral nervous system?
   1. Acetylcholine
   2. Norepinephrine
   3. Monoamine oxidase
   4. Choline
      A. 1. and 2.
      B. 1., 2., and 3.
      C. 3. and 4.
      D. All of the above

117. Which nervous system is responsible for involuntary body functions?
 A. Somatic nervous system
 B. Autonomic nervous system
 C. Central nervous system
 D. Brain stem

118. Which structure of the brain contains the center for respirations?
 A. Cerebral cortex
 B. Thalamus
 C. Medulla
 D. Hypothalamus

119. The apneustic center and pneumotaxic center are two centers that affect respiration. In which structure of the brain are they located?
 A. Medulla
 B. Pons
 C. Midbrain
 D. Cerebellum

120. Which structure of the brain is responsible for the fluid and electrolyte balance?
 A. Medulla
 B. Pons
 C. Thalamus
 D. Hypothalamus

121. Which scoring system is used to evaluate the neonatal cardiopulmonary status?
 A. Silverman Score
 B. Young Score
 C. Apgar Score
 D. Clark Score

122. Which scoring system is used to evaluate the level of respiratory distress in a neonate?
 A. Silverman Score
 B. Young Score
 C. Apgar Score
 D. Clark Score

123. What is the normal respiratory rate of a neonate?
    A. 80 to 100 breaths/min
    B. 60 to 80 breaths/ min
    C. 30 to 50 breaths/min
    D. 70 to 80 breaths/min

124. The average tidal volume of a neonate is
    A. 4 to 6 mL/kg
    B. 6 to 8 mL/kg
    C. 8 to 10 mL/kg
    D. 10 to 12 mL/kg

125. Fetal lung fluid is eliminated from the lung by which mechanism?
    A. Compression of the chest wall in the birth canal during the birth process
    B. Through the circulatory system by osmosis
    C. The lymphatic system
    D. All of the above

126. The first breath of the neonate is stimulated by
    1. the change in temperature between intrauterine and extrauterine conditions
    2. the rise in blood flow to the alveoli
    3. the bright lights and sounds in the delivery room
    4. the hypoxemia, acidemia, and hypercapnia that develop during the birth process
        A. 1. and 4.
        B. 4. only
        C. 1., 3., and 4.
        D. All of the above

127. The intrathoracic pressure that must be generated to initiate the first breath is
    A. -10 to -50 cm H_2O
    B. -40 to -90 cm H_2O
    C. -60 to -120 cm H_2O
    D. Greater than -120 cm H_2O

128. An Apgar Score of 7 to 10 would indicate
  A. full cardiopulmonary resuscitation should be initiated
  B. mild to moderate asphyxia
  C. few, if any, supportive measures are needed
  D. moderate respiratory distress

129. Nasal continuous positive airway pressure (CPAP) without the use of endotracheal intubation in a neonate is possible due to
  A. neonate breathing only through the nasal passage
  B. the neonatal larynx is funnel-shaped, whereas the diameter of the adult larynx is more or less constant.
  C. the size of the tongue in relation to the size of the oral cavity
  D. All of the above

130. Maintenance of body heat in a neonate is a significant problem due to
  A. the size of body surface area
  B. 80% of body weight being water
  C. the skin of a neonate playing a much greater role in water and heat balance than that of an adult
  D. All of the above

131. When performing artificial ventilation on a neonate without an endotracheal tube
  A. maximum head tilt maneuver should be performed
  B. the head should be maintained in a neutral position
  C. the jaw thrust maneuver should be used
  D. a towel should be placed under the head

Explanatory Answers

34. D. As air passes through the nasal cavity it is filtered for particulate material by small strands of hair called cilia. These transport the foreign material toward the external nares for discharge. Finally, the air is warmed and humidified to 100% relative humidity. (**Ref.** 4, p. 7)

35. B. Just past the nasal cavity is the region of the pharynx. This is divided into three regions: the nasopharynx, oropharynx, and laryngopharynx. The larynx lies between the pharynx and trachea. (**Ref.** 4, p. 7)

36. C. The trachea for an average adult is approximately 12 cm long. This can also be expressed as 4.5 to 5.5 in. (1 in. = 2.54 cm) (**Ref.** 4, p. 8)

37. B. The diameter of an adult trachea averages 1.5 to 2.5 cm. (**Ref.** 5, p. 8)

38. B. The trachea is supported by a series of 16 to 20 C-shaped cartilaginous rings embedded in the front and sides with smooth muscle separating the trachea and esophagus. (**Ref.** 4, p. 7)

39. C. The trachea extends from the larynx to the subdivisions of the left and right main stem bronchi. The laryngopharynx lies superior to the trachea and the bronchioles are distal to the main stems and have a diameter less than 1 mm. (**Ref.** 4, p. 8)

40. A. Inspiration is initiated primarily by the diaphragm, with the abdominal, intercostal, and accessory muscles generally becoming functional during periods of stress. (**Ref.** 4, p. 12)

41. C. The lungs are surrounded by a layer of squamous epithelial tissue called the visceral pleura. The pneumo and thorax pleura do not exist. (**Ref.** 1, p. 223)

42. A. The layer of tissue separating the visceral pleura from the chest wall is called the parietal pleura. Between the visceral and parietal pleuras is a thin film of fluid occupying what is called the intrapleura space. (**Ref.** 1, p. 223)

43. A. The left lung consists of the left upper and left lower lobes. (**Ref.** 4, p. 9)

44. B. The right lung is divided into the right upper, right middle, and right lower lobes. (**Ref.** 4, p. 9)

45. D. Anatomical deadspace consists of all structures beginning with the nose and extending to the terminal bronchioles, including the pharynx, trachea, and main stem bronchi. (**Ref.** 4, p. 11)

46. B. There are approximately 300,000,000 alveoli within the thoracic cavity. Stretched out this would occupy the surface of an entire tennis court. (**Ref.** 1, p. 224)

47. A. There are approximately 16 generations or subdivisions of bronchioles extendings from the main stem to the terminal bronchioles. (**Ref.** 5, p. 10)

48. C. The rib cage is composed of 12 pairs of ribs. (**Ref.** 4, p. 12)

49. B. The first 7 pairs of ribs or "true ribs" are attached to the sternum by the costal cartilage. Ribs 8, 9, and 10 are adjoined to each preceding rib by cartilage. Ribs 11 and 12 are floating ribs and are embedded within the abdominal musculature. (**Ref.** 4, p. 12)

50. C. External ventilation describes the exchanges of oxygen for carbon dioxide within the alveolus. Internal respiration relates to the exchange of gas in the tissues. (**Ref.** 4, p. 8)

51. A. Tachypnea is described as rapid shallow breathing above normal ratio for an adult (12 to 18) (**Ref.** 4, p. 13; **Ref.** 5, p. 291)

52. A. Trepopnea is defined as breathing that is more comfortable in a particular position. (**Ref.** 4, p. 13)

53. B. Biot's ventilation describes short rapid breathing interrupted by pauses of 10 to 30 sec. This may be exhibited in cases of meningitis. (**Ref.** 4, p. 13)

54. C. Cheyne–Stokes' respirations correspond to cyclical breathing with gradual increasing and decreasing depths of respiration and apneic periods ranging from 5 to 30 sec. (**Ref.** 4, p. 13)

55. B. Dyspnea represents the patient's subjective description of labored or distressed respiration. (**Ref.** 4, p. 13)

56. C. The absence of dyspnea is described as normal spontaneous respiration between 12 and 18 breaths/min for a normal adult. (**Ref.** 4, p. 13)

57. B. An increased depth of ventilation is described as hyperpnea. (**Ref.** 4, p. 13)

58. C. Hyperventilation describes breathing in excess of that required to maintain P_{CO_2} (40 mmHg) and pH (7.40) at normal levels. P_{CO_2} will decrease while pH will increase. (**Ref.** 4, p. 13)

59. A. Hypoventilation is breaths at a rate or depth below that which is required to maintain normal P_{CO_2} and pH. P_{CO_2} will increase, pH will decrease. (**Ref.** 4, p. 13)

60. A. Kussmaul's respirations, often associated with diabetic keto acidosis, are described as shortness of breath occurring spasmodically (air hunger). (**Ref.** 4, p. 13)

61. A. Breathing of small volume as slowed breathing is termed oligopnea. (**Ref.** 4, p. 13)

62. A. Orthopnea is the inability to breathe unless in the upright position. It is often described as one, two, or three pillow orthopnea. This is based on how many pillows a patient usually props up while sleeping. (**Ref.** 4, p. 13)

63. A. Polypnea defines rapid breathing; however, it should be noted that often this is interchangeable with tachypnea. (**Ref.** 4, p. 13)

64. A. Painful breathing is termed ponopnea. Apnea describes the absence of spontaneous respirations. (**Ref. 4**, p. 13)

65. B. The exchange of oxygen and carbon dioxide occurs with the alveolar atria and respiratory bronchioles. These structures are collectively referred to as the respiratory unit Lobule. No gas exchange occurs within the terminal bronchioles. (**Ref. 4**, p. 8)

66. B. The exchange of gas between the vasculature and the tissues that it supplies is referred to as internal respiration. (**Ref. 4**, p. 8)

67. B. Humidity is defined as the amount of water contained within a gas. Relative humidity is defined as the amount of water within a gas divided by the maximum possible amount of water a gas can hold at a specific temperature. It is known that under the conditions of 100% relative humidity and a temperature of 37°C, one cubic meter of air can hold 43.8 grams of water. (**Ref. 4**, p. 129)

68. C. Hematocyte is a blood corpuscle. Hemolysis is the destruction of red blood cells with the liberation of hemoglobin which diffuses into the fluid surrounding them. Hemoglobin is a chromoprotein of red color. (**Ref. 2**, p. H-21)

69. A. The normal range is 37% to 47% with 41% being the normal value for an adult female. (**Ref. 2**, p. H-21)

70. B. The normal range is 40% to 54% with 45% being the normal value for an adult male. (**Ref. 2**, p. H-21)

71. D. Hemoglobin is the iron-containing pigment of the red blood cell. Hematocyte is a blood corpusle. Hemolysis is the destruction of red blood cells. Hematocrit is the percentage of total blood volume that consists of erythrocytes. (**Ref. 2**, p. H·21)

72. A. The average amount of hemoglobin in the adult male is 14 to 16 g/100 mL of blood. (**Ref. 2**, p. H-21)

73. A. The average range of hemoglobin for adult females is within the normal average for both males and females of 14 to 16 g/100 mL of blood. (**Ref. 2**, p. H-21)

74. A. The red cell count in males is approximately 5,400,000 cells/mm³ of blood. Muscular exercise and emotional states are associated with a temporary increase. Red blood cell production is stimulated by any factor lowering oxygen available to the bone marrow or body tissue. (**Ref.** 3, p. 308)

75. B. The red cell count in females is approximately 4,700,000 cells/mm³ of blood. Muscular exercise and emotional states are associated with a temporary increase. Red blood cell production is stimulated by any factor lowering oxygen available to the bone marrow or body tissue. (**Ref.** 3, p. 308)

76. D. Another name for red blood cells is erythrocytes. Macrophages are large cells which engulf cells and cellular debris. Thrombocytes or platelets provide thrombokinase for blood coagulation, leukocytes, or white cells which produce antibodies. (**Ref.** 3, p. 308)

77. B. Leukopenia is the reduction in the number of white blood cells, occurring occasionally in viral diseases. (**Ref.** 3, p. 311)

78. A. Macrophages are a type of white cell which engulf cells and cellular debris. Thrombocytes or platelets provide thrombokinese for blood coagulation. Erythrocytes are red blood cells. (**Ref.** 3, p. 309)

79. C. The total leukocyte count ranges from 5,000 to 10,000/mm³; however, it may be as low as 500,000 in leukemia. (**Ref.** 3, p. 311)

80. C. The T-wave represents repolarization of the ventricles. The P-wave delineates atrial depolarization, while the Q and R occur as a result of ventricular depolarization. (**Ref.** 5, p. 32)

81. A. The term bigeminy is used when an abnormal ventricular beat (PVC) is coupled to a normal sinus beat. Ventricular tachycardia refers to a ventricular rate greater than 100 beats/min. Eventually this can deteriorate into ventricular fibrillation (ineffective contraction), which is life-threatening. (**Ref.** 5, p. 36)

82. A. The SA (sino-atrial) node or pacemaker of the heart sends impulses to the AV node, which in turn conducts impulses through the bundle of His and eventually terminates in the Perkinje's fibers. (**Ref.** 5, p. 27)

83. D. All three separate mechanisms are involved in hemostasis, or checking the flow of blood. When a vessel larger than a capillary is cut or damaged, platelets accumulate at the site of injury and adhere to the vascular endothelium. Simultaneously, vasoconstriction of muscle-containing vessels occurs. The process of hemostasis is completed with the formation of a fibrin clot. (**Ref.** 3, p. 315)

84. B. Purpura refers to loss of blood with the subcutaneous tissue. Thrombosis is clotting in blood vessels. Hemophilia is a hereditary bleeding disease characterized by delayed coagulation of the blood. (**Ref.** 3, p. 319)

85. A. Type O blood is a universal donor because O blood has no antigens. (**Ref.** 3, p. 314)

86. A. Type AB blood is a universal recipient because it has no antibodies. (**Ref.** 3, p. 314)

87. A. The osmotic pressure of human blood is maintained by electrolytes, sugar, plasma protein, and other crystalloids dissolved in plasma. (**Ref.** 3, p. 315)

88. D. The wall of the heart consists of three distinct layers, the epicardium, myocardium, and endocardium. (**Ref.** 3, p. 324)

89. C. The left ventricle walls are three times as thick as those of the right ventricle. (**Ref.** 3, p. 324)

90. C. The three veins emptying into the right atrium are: the inferior and superior venae cavae, bringing blood from the lower and upper portions of the body; with the coronary sinus draining blood from the heart itself. (**Ref.** 3, p. 324)

91. D. The pulmonary artery carries blood to the lungs and leaves from the superior surface of the right ventricle. (**Ref.** 3, p. 324)

92. A. Blood is forced from the left ventricle through the aorta to all parts of the body except the lungs. (**Ref.** 3, p. 324)

93. C. The left atrium receives blood from the four pulmonary veins draining oxygenated blood from the lungs. (**Ref.** 3, p. 324)

94. C. The tricuspid and mitral valves are the two atrioventricular valves which are thin, leaf-like structures located between the atrium and ventricles. (**Ref.** 3, p. 324)

95. B. The aortic valve is located at the attachment of the aorta to the left ventricle. (**Ref.** 3, p. 324)

96. B. The pulmonary artery is attached to the right ventricle and carries blood to the lungs. The pulmonary valve prevents retrograde flow into the right ventricle. (**Ref.** 3, p. 324)

97. B. If as long as 4 min is allowed to elapse, there can be irreversible damage to the brain. (**Ref.** 3, p. 336)

98. C. The walls of the heart consist of three distinct layers: the epicardium, myocardium, and endocardium. (**Ref.** 3, p. 320)

99. B. The foramen ovale is the opening between the two atria, permitting blood to flow from the right atrium into the left atrium. (**Ref.** 3, p. 338)

100. C. The ductus arteriosus is the blood vessel connecting the pulmonary artery to the aorta. The ductus venous is the vessel connecting the umbilical vein to the inferior vena cava. (**Ref.** 3, p. 338)

101. D. The initial stages of progressive shock are characterized by apprehension, cold skin, cyanosis of the fingertips, reduced blood pressure (most often), shallow respiratory activity, sweating, and rapid pulse. (**Ref.** 3, p. 373)

102. C. The average volume of blood ejected by the heart per beat is 60 to 70 mL. (**Ref.** 3, p. 335)

103. A. The inferior and superior venae cavae empty into the right atrium. (**Ref.** 13, p. 551)

104. B. The mitral valve is located between the left atrium and left ventricle. (**Ref.** 13, p. 555)

105. C. The tricuspid valve is located between the right atrium and right ventricle. (**Ref.** 13, p. 555)

106. C. Complete atrioventricular block (third degree block) represents a total dissociation of the atrial and ventricular rhythms. The ventricular sets its own rhythm in the atrioventricular node or in the bundle of His at a rate of 30 to 45 beats/min. At times, the rate is higher. (**Ref.** 3, p. 332)

107. A. In the first degree block, a delay in atrioventricular conduction occurs. The delay cannot be clinically recognized, but is indicated by a prolonged PR interval in the electrocardiogram. (**Ref.** 3, p. 332)

108. C. Cardiac rates less than 60 beats/min indicate a bradycardia. In the case of a sinus arrhythmia rates vary, but generally are between 60 and 100 beats/min as in a normal sinus rhythm. In sinus tachycardia, cardiac rates exceed 100 beats/min. (**Ref.** 22, p. 263)

109. B. Both sinus arrhythmias and normal rhythms vary between 60 and 100 beats/min. Sinus bradycardias are less than 60 beats/min. Sinus tachycardias denote rates greater than 100 beats/min. (**Ref.** 22, p. 264)

110. B. Somas are the site for the synthesis of transmitter substance. Dendrites carry impulses to the cell body, while axons carry impulses away from cell bodies. (**Ref.** 22, p. 142)

111. C. Axons carry impulses away from cell bodies. Only one axon usually arises from a cell body. Each neuron may contain 10,000 dendrites which carry impulses to the cell body innervating the soma to synthesize transmitter substances. (**Ref.** 22, p. 142)

112. A. Sensory (also known as afferent) neurons transmit impulses to the brain. Motor or effector neurons relay impulses to muscles. Interneurons are the conducting pathways between sensory and motor neurons. (**Ref.** 22, p. 142)

113. B. The nerve synapse is the junction between one neuron, another neuron, muscle, or gland. Impulses leaving an axon of one neuron are transmitted across these synapses through a chemical process to other neurons, muscles, or glands to achieve a specific effect, i.e., contraction of muscles, etc. (**Ref.** 22, p. 143)

114. C. Norepinephrine and acetylcholine are substances synthesized within the neuron that facilitate transmission from one nerve to another. They are known as transmitter substances. Acidosis decreases the ability of these substances to transfer across a synapse. (**Ref.** 22, p. 145)

115. B. Alkalosis enhances the ability of norepinephrine and acetylcholine to be transmitted across synaptic junctions. (**Ref.** 22, p. 145)

116. A. Both acetylcholine and norepinephrine are synthesized within the neuron and act as transmitter substances. Monoamine oxidase is the enzyme responsible for the breakdown of norepinephrine. Choline is the by-product of the breakdown of acetylcholine. (**Ref.** 22, p. 145)

117. B. If you think of autonomic as automatic, you can remember that this nervous system is responsible for involuntary functions. Conversely, the somatic system is responsible for voluntary bodily function. The brain stem is a subdivision of the central nervous system. (**Ref.** 22, p. 147)

118. C. The portion of the brain that controls respiration is the medulla. It lies within the brain stem itself. The cerebral cortex is responsible for all higher brain functions such as memory and reasoning. The thalamus and hypothalamus lie between the cortex and the brain stem, with the thalamus being primarily responsible for sensatory function and the hypothalamus being responsible for hormonal control as well as vegetative functions (eating, sleeping, sexual behavior). (**Ref.** 22, p. 148)

119. B. The pons, also located in the brain stem, contains the apneustic (inspiratory inhibitor) and pneumotaxic (sustained inspiration) centers. These centers working in conjunction result in rhythmic ventilation. The midbrain controls audio and visual senses while the cerebellum is responsible for fine motor activity. (**Ref.** 22, p. 149)

120. D. The hypothalamus, innervated by the autonomic nervous system, controls fluid and electrolyte balance as well as temperature, emotional, and behavioral regulation. The medulla and pons coordinate respiration while the thalamus is the primary relay station for hearing, touch, pressure, and pain. (**Ref.** 22, p. 148)

121. C. The Apgar Score, done at 1 and 5 min after birth, is a system to evaluate neonates as well as all infants initially after birth. Scaling is done between 0 and 10, and is based on heart rate, respiratory rate, color, tone, and response to stimulation. The Silverman Score evaluates degree of respiratory distress. (**Ref.** 22, p. 171)

122. A. The Silverman Score is also a scale of 0 to 10, measuring the degree of respiratory distress. It is based on retractions, chest movement, grunting, and nasal flaring. Apgar measures cardiopulmonary status. Young and Clark scores are fictitious. (**Ref.** 22, p. 172)

123. C. Normal respiratory rate for neonates is 2 to 3 times higher than the average adults (30 to 50 breaths/min). Higher respiratory rates are considered tachypnic. Generally, the more premature the neonate the higher the respiratory rate. (**Ref.** 22, p. 173)

124. B. The average tidal volume for a neonate is 6 to 8 mL/kg. (**Ref.** 22, p. 173)

125. D. Fetal lung fluid is eliminated in three ways. First, as the infant passes through the birth canal the pressure exerted on its chest wall forces some of this fluid out. Second, as pulmonary blood flow increases, since the fetal lung is low in protein, oncotic pressure draws some fluid into the pulmonary circulation. Lastly, the lymphatic system is responsible for absorption of excess fluid. (**Ref.** 22, p. 170)

126. C. Immediately after birth, factors such as bright lights and loud sounds, and the infant's skin being exposed to a drop in temperature, all stimulate the infant to take its first breath. More importantly, hypoxia and the acute drop in pH stimulate chemoreceptors to initiate that first breath. (**Ref.** 22, p. 170)

127. B. A pressure of -40 to -90 cmH$_2$O must be generated to initiate the first breath, after which inspiratory volume will exceed expiratory volume until the functional residual capacity is established. (**Ref.** 22, p. 171)

128. C. Few if any measures are needed for a score of 7 to 10. A score of 0 to 3 requires full cardiopulmonary resuscitation. A score of 4 to 6 is classified as mild to moderate asphyxia and usually requires suctioning, administration of oxygen, and possibly ventilation. (**Ref.** 22, p. 171)

129. C. Unless an infant is crying, most of his/her tidal volume is moved through the nasal passage due to the size of his/her tongue in relation to the oral cavity. (**Ref.** 22, p. 178)

130. D. The neonate's body surface area (BSA) is 9 times that of an adult in relation to its size. While an adult weight is only 60% water, the neonate is comprised of 80% water. Therefore, the thin skin membrane of the neonate with its large BSA allows evaporation of water causing difficulty maintaining body heat. (**Ref.** 22, p. 180)

131. B. Due to the cartilage comprising the neonate's trachea being flexible and not fully formed, hyperextension of the neck may cause compression of the airway and result in obstruction. Since you are ventilating a neonate's nose and mouth, jaw thrust is unnecessary. (**Ref.** 22, p. 179)

4 Hemodynamic Monitoring

DIRECTIONS (Questions 132–165): Each of the questions or incomplete statements below is followed by four suggested answers or completions. Select the **one** that is **best** in each case.

132. Central venous pressure (CVP) represents the
    A. subclavian vein pressure
    B. left atrial pressure
    C. right atrial pressure
    D. right ventricle pressure

133. Normal value for CVP in an adult is
    A. 0 to 8 mmHg
    B. 5 to 16 mmHg
    C. 8 to 20 mmHg
    D. 15 to 28 mmHg

134. The normal value of the mean pulmonary artery pressure is
    A. 0 to 8 mmHg
    B. 5 to 16 mmHg
    C. 8 to 20 mmHg
    D. 15 to 28 mmHg

135. The pulmonary wedge pressure (PWP) represents
    A. mean right atrial pressure
    B. mean pulmonary artery pressure
    C. mean left ventrical pressure
    D. mean left atrial pressure

46

136. The normal value for PWP in adults is
    A. 0 to 8 mmHg
    B. 2 to 12 mmHg
    C. 5 to 16 mmHg
    D. 10 to 22 mmHg

137. The Fick equation is used to determine
    A. cardiac output
    B. pulmonary wedge pressure
    C. arterial oxygen content
    D. mixed venous oxygen content

138. The normal cardiac index is
    A. 2.5 to 4 L/min/m^2
    B. 4 to 7 L/min/m^2
    C. 6 to 10 L/min/m^2
    D. 10 to 15 L/min/m^2

139. The Fick equation is
    A. total 0_2 available $= (Q) \times (Ca_{O_2})$
    B. $V_{O_2} = (Q) \times (Ca_{O_2} - Cv_{O_2})$
    C. $Q = V_{O_2} \times (Ca_{O_2} - Cv_{O_2})$
    D. PWP $= (PAP-LAP) \times (Q)$

140. Which is incorrect about the Swan–Ganz catheter?
    A. Uses thermal dilution method
    B. Uses dye dilution
    C. The proximal port usually lies in the right atrium
    D. Used to measure cardiac output

141. The normal systolic pulmonary blood pressure in the adult
    is
    A. 0 to 8 mmHg
    B. 5 to 16 mmHg
    C. 10 to 22 mmHg
    D. 15 to 28 mmHg

142. The normal diastolic pulmonary arterial blood pressure in the adult is
    A. 0 to 8 mmHg
    B. 5 to 16 mmHg
    C. 10 to 22 mmHg
    D. 15 to 28 mmHg

143. The normal pulmonary vascular resistance is
    A. 2 mmHg/L/min
    B. 5 mmHg/L/min
    C. 10 mmHg/L/min
    D. 17 mmHg/L/min

144. The pulmonary artery pressure (PAP)
    A. assesses right ventricular function
    B. assesses pulmonary arterial resistance
    C. is directly measured
    D. all of the above

145. If the left ventricle is not pumping adequately, the PWP will
    A. increase
    B. decrease
    C. remain the same
    D. none of the above

146. The formula used in calculating systemic vascular resistance is
    A. $R = (MAP - \overline{RAP})/Q$
    B. $R = (PAP - LAP)/Q$
    C. $R = (PAP - PWP)/Q$
    D. $R = (PAP - CVP)/Q$

147. The normal systemic vascular resistance equals
    A. 2 mmHg/L/min
    B. 5 mmHg/L/min
    C. 10 mmHg/L/min
    D. 17 mmHg/L/min

148. The normal mean pulmonary arterial pressure is
   A. 5 mmHg
   B. 30 mmHg
   C. 10 to 22 mmHg
   D. 0 to 7 mmHg

149. Cardiac output is equal to the product of the pulse rate and
   A. mean atrial pressure
   B. diastolic filling period
   C. stroke volume
   D. hemoglobin level

150. Cardiac output is determined by which of the following factors?
   1. Ventricular end-diastolic volume
   2. Myocardial contractility
   3. Ventricular afterload
   4. Heart rate
      A. 1. and 2.
      B. 1., 2., and 3.
      C. 1. and 3.
      D. All of the above

151. The normal upper limit pressure of the right atrium during right heart catherization is
   A. 8 mmHg
   B. 10 mmHg
   C. 15 mmHg
   D. 7 mmHg

152. A pulmonary artery catheter may be inserted into the right heart through which of the following?
   1. Internal jugular
   2. Basilic
   3. Subclavian
   4. Femoral veins
      A. 3. and 4.
      B. 2., 3., and 4.
      C. 2. and 3.
      D. All of the above

153. The small inflatable balloon located at the end of the pulmonary artery catheter is filled with
    A. helium
    B. nitrogen
    C. oxygen
    D. air

154. The pulmonary artery catheter has two lumens. One terminates in the pulmonary artery. The second, when the catheter is properly positioned, ends where?
    A. Pulmonary artery
    B. Right atrium
    C. Right ventricle
    D. Left atrium

155. A ventricle is stated to be noncompliant if
    A. it can accept a large volume of blood with only a small rise in pressure
    B. it can accept a large volume of blood with a slight rise in pressure
    C. the pressure rises sharply as volume increases
    D. none of the above

156. The volume of blood present in the RV at end diastole is called
    A. RV preload
    B. RV afterload
    C. Stroke volume
    D. RV index

157. The mean value of the pulmonary arterial wedge pressure (PAWP) reflects the mean
    A. right ventricle pressure
    B. left ventricle pressure
    C. right atrium pressure
    D. left atrium pressure

158. Which of the following is incorrect about pulmonary arterial catheters?
   A. Persistent wedging may lead to pulmonary infarction
   B. Fluid must be used to inflate the balloon
   C. Fluid should never be flushed through the catheter under high pressure when it is in the wedged position
   D. The balloon should not be overinflated

159. A complication of inserting the pulmonary arterial catheter at the subclavian is
   A. fluoroscopy often required
   B. excessive bleeding
   C. pneumothorax
   D. all of the above

160. Which of the following are indicators of increased risk of pulmonary complications in the preoperative patient?
   1. FEF 25% to 75% < 1.2 L/sec or 40% predicted
   2. Peak flow < 200 L/min
   3. MVV $< 50\%$ predicted
   4. Arterial $P_{CO_2} > 46$ mmHg
      A. 1. and 2.
      B. 2. only
      C. 1., 2., and 4.
      D. All of the above

161. Which of the following is incorrect about peak expiratory flow rates?
   A. The peak flow rate is markedly affected by obstruction of large airways
   B. Flow rates of less than 400 L/min suggest impaired cough efficiency
   C. It provides a valuable tool for quickly identifying gross pulmonary disability
   D. Normal values in healthy males under 40 years of age are greater than 500 L/min

162. In the postpneumonectomy patient, which of the following values would the clinician expect to see?
    A. FVC, FEV_1 (L) normal $FEV_1/FVC\%$
    B. FVC, FEV_1 (L) $FEV_1/FVC\%$
    C. FVC, FEV_1 (L) $FEV_1/FVC\%$
    D. FVC, FEV_1, normal $FEV_1/FVC\%$

163. The normal maximal static expiratory pressure (PE max) is
    A. +100 cm H_2O
    B. +150 cm H_2O
    C. +200 cm H_2O
    D. none of the above

164. A PE max of less than +40 cm H_2O suggests
    A. inability to take a deep breath
    B. severely impaired coughing ability
    C. obstructive airway disease
    D. restrictive airway disease

165. A pneumonectomy should not be allowed unless the predicted postoperative FEV_1 is
    A. at least 800 ml
    B. at least 1000 ml
    C. one-half of the preoperative achieved value
    D. none of the above

Explanatory Answers

132. C. The central venous pressure is measured directly through a catheter whose tip lies within the right atrium. It is a good indicator of blood volume and right ventricular preload. Left atrial pressure can only be determined with a Swan–Ganz catheter. Subclavian vein pressure does not reflect total venous blood volume. (**Ref.** 22, p. 231)

133. A. The normal value for CVP in the adult is 0 to 8 mmHg. Anything higher is abnormal and may represent volume overload or right-sided heart failure. (**Ref.** 22, p. 234)

134. C. Mean pulmonary artery pressure is used as an indicator of resistance to which the right ventricle must pump against. Its normal value ranges from 10 to 22 mmHg. The lower that number, the less work on the right ventricle; the higher, the more work inflicted on the right ventricle. (**Ref.** 22, p. 234)

135. D. Essentially, pulmonary wedge pressure represents mean left atrial pressure. More commonly it is associated with left ventricular preload or the left ventricular end diastolic pressure. Since this pressure is measured distal to a balloon occluding a branch of the pulmonary artery, right-sided pressures have no bearing on the measurement. (**Ref.** 22, p. 234)

136. B. Normal pulmonary wedge pressures (PWP) in adults is 2 to 12 mmHg. Lower pressures might indicate poor volume, while higher pressures (> 18 mmHg) may indicate left ventricular failure. Pressures above 20 to 25 mmHg may precipitate pulmonary edema. (**Ref.** 22, p. 235)

137. A. The Fick equation is used to determine cardiac output. Although pulmonary wedge pressures are affected by cardiac output it is not a linear determinant. Arterial oxygen and mixed venous oxygen contents are factors of the Fick equation. (**Ref.** 22, p. 236)

138. A. Since cardiac outputs vary between people in terms of body size, a more accurate expression is the cardiac index. It is determined from cardiac output in L/min per body surface area in square meters. The normal value is 2.5 to 4 L/min/m². Anything higher indicates a high cardiac output. Anything less indicates a low cardiac output. (**Ref.** 22, p. 239)

139. B. The Fick equation is expressed as

$$Vo_2 = (Q) \times (Cao_2 - Cvo_2)$$

By solving for Vo_2 cardiac output can be determined by

$$Q = \frac{Vo_2}{A - Vo_2}$$

(**Ref.** 22, p. 236)

140. B. Swan–Ganz catheters measure cardiac output (C.O.) by thermal dilution. A solution with a known volume and temperature is injected into the proximal port while a thermister at the distal end plots changes in temperature over time to determine C.O. The proximal port lies within the right atrium to measure CVP pressures. The dye dilution requires a CVP or pulmonary artery catheter as well as an additional catheter located in a major systemic artery. (**Ref.** 22, p. 238)

141. D. Normal systolic pulmonary blood pressure in adults is 15 to 28 mmHg. 0 to 8 mmHg represents CVP pressures. 5 to 16 mmHg represents diastolic pulmonary artery pressures. 10 to 22 mmHg represents mean pulmonary artery pressures. In general, systolic pulmonary artery blood pressure represents right ventricular function. (**Ref.** 22, p. 234)

142. B. The normal diastolic pulmonary arterial blood pressure is 5 to 16 mmHg and is a function of pulmonary arterial resistance. It also is used to reflect left atrial pressure in the absence of mitral stenosis or mitral regurgitation. (**Ref.** 22, p. 234)

143. A. The equation for pulmonary vascular resistance equals $(\overline{PAP} - \overline{LAP})/\dot{Q}$, where $\overline{PAP}$ = mean pulmonary arterial pressure; $\overline{LAP}$ = mean left atrial pressure; $\dot{Q}$ = cardiac output. Substituting normal values results in the equal of $(16 - 6)$ mmHg/ 5 L/min = 2 mmHg/L/min. (**Ref.** 22, p. 234)

144. D. The pulmonary artery pressure is directly measured via a pulmonary arterial catheter and assesses right ventricular function (systolic) and pulmonary arterial resistance (diastolic). (**Ref.** 22, p. 236)

145. A. If the left ventricle is not pumping adequately, the PWP will increase. Since the PWP is a pressure measured distal to the pulmonary artery, it is a reflection of back pressure from the left side of the heart. The more back pressure, the higher the PWP, thus left-sided heart failure. (**Ref.** 22, p. 233)

146. A. The formula for systemic vascular resistance (SVR) is:

$$SVR = \frac{MAP - \overline{RAP}}{\text{cardiac output}}$$

where MAP = mean arterial pressure, and $\overline{RAP}$ = mean right atrial pressure. Answer B. represents the formula for pulmonary vascular resistance. Answers C. and D. are fictitious. (**Ref.** 22, p. 234)

147. D. Substituting normal values for the equation (See Answer 146)

$$SVR = \frac{MAP - \overline{RAP}}{\text{cardiac output}}$$

$$SVR = \frac{(90 - 5) \text{ mmHg}}{5 \text{ L/min}} = \frac{17 \text{ mmHg}}{\text{L/min}}$$

148. C. The normal mean pulmonary arterial blood pressure is 10 to 22 mmHg. It is used to assess the resistance that the right ventricle must pump against. (**Ref.** 22, p. 235)

149. C. Cardiac output is equal to the product of the pulse rate and stroke volume. (**Ref.** 27, p. 12)

150. D. Cardiac output is determined by four independent but interrelated factors: ventricular end diastolic volume, myocardial contractility, ventricular afterload, and heart rate. (**Ref.** 27, p. 12)

151. A. The normal upper limit pressure of the right atrium during right heart catheterization is 8 mmHg. (**Ref.** 27, p. 13)

152. D. Access to the right heart is achieved through the internal jugular, basilic, subclavian, or femoral veins. (**Ref.** 27, p. 13)

153. D. A small inflatable balloon located at the distal end of the catheter is filled with approximately 1.5 mL of air and floats through the RA and RV into the RA as the catheter is advanced. (**Ref.** 27, p. 13)

154. B. The pulmonary artery has two lumens. One terminates in the pulmonary artery. The second, when the catheter is properly positioned, ends in the right atrium. (**Ref.** 27, p. 14)

155. C. The change in right ventricle pressure as its volume increases is related to ventricular compliance: a ventricle that can accept a large volume of blood with only a small rise in pressure is compliant, but if the pressure rises sharply as ventricular volume increases, the ventricle is noncompliant. (**Ref.** 27, p. 14)

156. A. The volume of blood present in the RV at end diastole is called the RV preload. (**Ref.** 27, p. 14)

157. D. The mean value of the pulmonary arterial wedge pressure reflects mean left atrial pressure, as long as nothing obstructs the flow of blood from the pulmonary arteriolar bed to the left atrium. (**Ref.** 27, p. 14)

158. B. Care must be taken during wedge pressure recording. Overinflation of the balloon may lead to "overwedging," in which the recorded pressure is far in excess of the actual PAWP. The catheter must never be left in wedged position for more than 1 minute, since this may lead to pulmonary infarction. Fluid must never be used to inflate the balloon. Finally, fluid should never be flushed through the catheter under high pressure when it is in the wedged position. (**Ref.** 27, p. 14)

159. C. A complication of subclavian puncture while inserting the pulmonary arterial catheter is pneumothorax. (**Ref.** 27, p. 14)

160. D. Indicators of increased risk of pulmonary complications in the preoperative patient include: $FEV_1 < 2.0$ L; FEF 25% to 75% < 1.2 L/sec or $< 40\%$ predicted; peak flow < 200 L/min, MVV $< 50\%$ predicted; arterial $Pco_2 > 46$ mmHg and sputum volume > 60 mL/day. (**Ref.** 29, p. 168)

161. B. Peak expiratory flow rates of < 200 L/min suggest impaired cough efficiency and significant postoperative respiratory complications. (**Ref.** 29, p. 169)

162. D. In the postpneumonectomy patient, a clinician would expect to see a decrease in the FVC, a decrease in FEV_1 and a normal $FEV_1/FVC\%$. (**Ref.** 29, p. 169)

163. C. The maximal static expiratory pressure (PE max) is measured when expiratory muscles are optimally stretched after a full inspiration to near total lung capacity. They are useful in evaluating patients with neuromuscular disease. The normal value is $+200$ cm H_2O. (**Ref.** 29, p. 169)

164. B. A PE max of less than $+40$ cm H_2O suggests severely impaired coughing ability. (**Ref.** 29, p. 169)

165. A. A predicted postoperative FEV_1 of at least 800 mL is required before allowing pneumonectomy because significant resting carbon dioxide retention occurs with lower values. (**Ref.** 29, p. 171)

5 Pharmacology

DIRECTIONS (Questions 166–188): Each of the questions or incomplete statements below is followed by four suggested answers or completions. Select the **one** that is **best** in each case.

---

166. Digitalis affects the cardiac function through which of the following mechanisms?
    1. Increases the strength of the myocardial contraction
    2. Slows the heart rate
    3. Lowers the blood pressure
    4. Increases the blood pressure
        A. 1. and 2.
        B. 1., 2., and 3.
        C. 1., 2., and 4.
        D. 1. only

167. Which of the following are the most common effects seen on the EKG tracing or monitor with therapeutic doses of digitalis?
    A. S–T segment depression
    B. P–R interval lengthening
    C. Peaked P-wave
    D. T-wave inversion

168. Repeated prothrombin time determinations are required with administration of
   A. dicumarol
   B. heprin
   C. vitamin K
   D. protamine

169. Heprin therapy is regulated by determining the patient's
   A. prothrombin time
   B. clotting time
   C. platelet count
   D. bleeding time

170. Which of the following factors impair drug metabolism?
   1. Age
   2. Cardiac failure
   3. Renal insufficiency
   4. Cigarette smoking
      A. 1. and 4.
      B. 2. and 3.
      C. 1., 3., and 4.
      D. All of the above

171. What does the pharmacological abbreviation "a.c." mean?
   A. By mouth
   B. After meals
   C. Before meals
   D. Immediately

172. Which of the following abbreviations means "with"?
   A. ā
   B. aq
   C. s̄
   D. c̄

173. Which of the following abbreviations means "without"?
   A. ā
   B. aq
   C. s̄
   D. c̄

174. Which of the following abbreviations means "drop(s)"?
   A. gtt
   B. aq
   C. qs
   D. supp

175. Which of the following abbreviations means "after meals"?
   A. qs
   B. s.c.
   C. p.c.
   D. h.s.

176. The "drop" so often used in prescribing inhalation solutions is a very imprecise measurement. Which of the following factors influence the volume?
   1. Viscosity of the solution
   2. Temperature and consistency of the solution
   3. Construction of the dropper
   4. Whether the dropper is in vertical position
      A. 1. and 2.
      B. 1. only
      C. None of the above
      D. All of the above

177. The drug diazepam
   A. causes significant respiratory depression in normal patients
   B. reduces minute ventilation only slightly when hypnotic doses are administered
   C. can cause alveolar hypoventilation and respiratory acidosis in patients with COPD
   D. is not additive in its respiratory depression

178. The drug doxapram
   A. is a potent respiratory depressant
   B. stimulates the peripheral respiratory receptors only
   C. causes increase in both respiratory rate and tidal volume
   D. is used in treatment of acute respiratory failure in patients with COPD

179. Progestins
   A. cause hyperventilation and an elevated end-tidal CO_2
   B. have been used to treat sleep apnea and COPD with some success
   C. stimulate central respiratory centers only
   D. are antianalgesic

180. Halothane, a known bronchodilator, is considered the anesthetic of choice for COPD patients. The side effect is
   A. circulatory depression
   B. hypertension
   C. arrhythmias
   D. A. and C.

181. Albuterol administered preoperatively by metered aerosol (1 to 4 puffs) should prove effective against bronchospasm for
   A. 2 h
   B. 4 h
   C. 6 h
   D. 8 h

182. The drug of choice to treat legionellosis is
   A. penicillin
   B. erythromycin
   C. cephalosporin
   D. aminoglycoside

183. Recombivax-HB and Hepravax-B are two vaccines used to immunize against
   A. influenza
   B. polio
   C. hepatitis B
   D. AIDS

184. The onset of action of beta agonists by either the inhalation of parenteral routes is usually within what time frame?
   A. 15 to 20 min
   B. 5 to 10 min
   C. 20 to 30 min
   D. 30 to 40 min

185. Which of the following beta agonists stimulate both beta-1 and beta-2 receptors?
 1. Epinephrine
 2. Isoproterenol
 3. Isoetharine
 4. Metaproterenol
   A. 1. and 2.
   B. 1., 3., and 4.
   C. 1., 2., and 4.
   D. 2. only

186. The therapeutic range of blood levels for theophylline is
   A. 5 to 10 μg/mL
   B. 10 to 20 μg/mL
   C. 15 to 25 μg/mL
   D. 30 to 40 μg/mL

187. The frequently recommended loading dose of aminophylline is
   A. 2 to 3 mg/kg
   B. 4 to 5 mg/kg
   C. 5 to 6 mg/kg
   D. 8 to 10 mg/kg

188. What percentage of the total dose of medication placed in a compressor-driven nebulizer is delivered to the lungs?
   A. 10% to 15%
   B. 20% to 25%
   C. 30% to 35%
   D. Greater than 50%

Explanatory Answers

166. A. Digitalis affects cardiac functions through two important mechanisms: (1) Digitalis has positive inotropic actium. It influences the mechanical performance of the heart by increasing the strength of myocardial contraction. (2) Digitalis alters the electric behavior of heart muscle through its actions on myocardial automaticity, conduction velocity, and refractory period. (**Ref.** 15, p. 142)

167. B. Conduction velocity is decreased with all concentrations of digitalis. The atrioventricular conduction system is particularly affected. This slowing of conduction is partly caused by the direct action of digitalis, but mostly by an increase in vagal action and a decrease in adrenergic action. This is shown on the electrocardiogram by a prolonged P–R interval. (**Ref.** 15, p. 193)

168. A. Repeated prothrombin time determinations are required with administration of dicumarol. (**Ref.** 15, p. 190)

169. B. Heparin prevents coagulation by (1) interfering with the formation of thrombin from prothrombin, (2) preventing thrombin from acting as a catalyst in converting fibrinogen into fibrin, and (3) preventing agglutination and disintegration of platelets and releasing their thromboplastin. Therefore, heparin increases clotting time in blood. (**Ref.** 15, p. 187)

170. D. Young and elderly patients will metabolize certain drugs more slowly. Patients in cardiac failure may not metabolize drugs as expected depending on the degree of failure. Drug toxicity may develop in patients with renal or hepatic insufficiency. Patients can metabolize drugs such as theophylline more rapidly if they use tobacco. (**Ref.** 16, p. 17)

171. C. The abbreviation a.c. refers to "before meals"; p.o. is "by mouth"; p.c. is "after meals"; and stat is "immediate." (**Ref.** 16, p. 37)

172. D. c̄ stands for "with"; ā means "before"; aq is synonymous with "water"; and s̄ is "without." (**Ref.** 16, p. 37)

173. C. s̄ is "without." (**Ref.** 16, p. 37)

174. A. The abbreviation for "drop(s)" is gtt; aq is the standard abbreviation for "water"; q.s. refers to the amount which is sufficient; and supp indicates "suppository." (**Ref.** 16, p. 37)

175. C. The accepted abbreviation for "before meals" is p.c.; s.q. refers to "subcutaneous"; and h.s. means "at bedtime." (**Ref.** 16, p. 37)

176. D. The more viscous a solution, the greater the size of the drop it will produce. Other variables affecting droplet size include temperature, consistency of the solution, construction of the dropper, and the position dropper is held in when fluid is expelled. (**Ref.** 16, p. 38)

177. B. Diazepam alone has few respiratory depressant effects. Minute volume and response to hypoxemia are slightly reduced. However, in patients with COPD or in conjunction with other CNS depressant drugs, diazepam may produce severe respiratory depression. (**Ref.** 21, p. 109)

178. D. Doxapram is a potent respiratory stimulant with a narrow therapeutic-to-toxic level. Therefore, its uses today are rare. However, it may still be indicated for patients in acute respiratory failure with COPD. It acts by stimulating both the central and peripheral respiratory receptors. (**Ref.** 21, p. 110)

179. B. Progestins have been used to stimulate larger tidal volumes in patients with sleep apnea, COPD, and difficult-to-wean patients. The mechanism or site of action remains unknown. Its discovery occurred when it was noted that during pregnancy women hyperventilated and demonstrated a decreased end-tidal CO_2 (**Ref.** 21, p. 111)

180. D. Circulatory depression and arrhythmias are known side effects to the administration of halothane. Hypotension may occur should excessive amounts of anesthetic be administered. (**Ref.** 30, p. 29)

181. C. Preoperative administration of albuterol may provide up to 6 h of bronchodilation. (**Ref.** 30, p. 29)

182. B. Penicillin, cephalosporins, and aminoglycosides thus far have demonstrated little effectiveness in the treatment of legionellosis. Erythromycin remains the antibiotic of choice. Its success has been attributed to its ability to enter the alveolar macrophage. (**Ref.** 37, p. 4)

183. C. Recombivax-HB and Hepravax-B are recommended for vaccination against hepatitis B. Hepravax-B is obtained from the plasma of known hepatitis B carriers while Recombivax-HB is developed from bread yeast. (**Ref.** 38, p. 85)

184. B. Onset of action for beta agonists by the parenteral or inhalational route is usually 5 to 10 min, although peak action may not occur for 20 to 30 min. (**Ref.** 35, p. 63)

185. A. Naturally occuring catecholamines such as epinephrine or isoproterenol stimulate both beta-1 and beta-2 receptors. Therefore, they have a higher incidence of cardiac side effects than beta-2 specific agents such as isoetharine or metaproterenol. (**Ref.** 35, p. 63)

186. B. The therapeutic level for theophylline is 10 to 20 μg/mL. Levels less than 10 μg/mL produce submaximal bronchodilation while levels greater than 20 μg/mL are associated with systemic side effects manifested by nausea, tachycardia, irritability, or headaches. (**Ref.** 35, p. 64)

187. C. When aminophylline is to be administered intravenously a recommended loading dose of 5 to 6 mg/kg should be instituted over a period of 20 min. (**Ref.** 35, p. 64)

188. A. Only approximately 10% to 15% of the total dose administered by a compressor-driven nebulizer is deposited in the lungs. The remaining 85% to 90% is either exhaled, or deposited in the oropharynx or tubing. (**Ref.** 35, p. 66)

6 Microbiology and Decontamination

DIRECTIONS (Questions 189–205): Each group of questions below consists of a set of lettered items, followed by a list of numbered definitions. For each lettered item, select the correct numbered definition.

Questions 189–198:

A.	Aerobic	**F.**	Bacteremia
B.	Anaerobic	**G.**	Bacteria
C.	Antiseptic	**H.**	Commensalism
D.	Asepsis	**I.**	Pathogen
E.	Autoclave	**J.**	Phagocyte

189. Microscopic, unicellular plants containing no chlorophyll, which reproduce by binary fission.

190. A cell capable of ingesting bacteria or other foreign particles.

191. To live in an atmosphere containing oxygen.

192. A substance that prevents or arrests the growth or action of microorganisms, either by inhibiting their activity or by destroying them.

193. A device for sterilizing medical supplies and equipment by steam under pressure.

194. The presence of bacteria in blood; does not imply growth of bacteria.

195. Any disease-producing microorganism or material.

196. To live in an atmosphere without oxygen.

197. The state or condition of complete absence of all bacteria, an ideal state.

198. A symbiotic association between two organisms, causing no harm to either.

Questions 199–205:
    A. Bacilli
    B. Cocci
    C. Flora, resident
    D. Flora, transient
    E. Gram-negative organisms
    F. Gram-positive organisms
    G. Spirochetes

199. The bacteria on the surface of the skin, which can be easily removed by normal handwashing.

200. An organism that appears red as result of treatment with Gram's staining technique.

201. Bacteria that appear under the microscope as rods.

202. Slender, frexuous, or corkscrew-shaped organisms that are highly mobile.

203. The bacteria that reside below the surface of the skin, in the pore openings, and among the cracks, crevices, and folds of the skin. They cannot be removed by ordinary washing.

204. The bacteria appearing under the microscope as circles, dots, or spores.

205. An organism that appears blue as a result of treatment with Gram's staining technique.

DIRECTIONS (Questions 206–266): Each of the questions or incomplete statements below is followed by four suggested answers or completions. Select the **one** that is **best** in each case.

---

206. The process, physical or chemical, that will destroy all forms of life, including bacteria, mold, spores, and viruses is called
   A. sterilization
   B. sanitizer
   C. germicide
   D. fungicide

207. The chemical agent that destroys disease germs (kills growing forms) or other harmful microorganisms, but not necessarily the resistant spore forms, is a
   A. disinfectant
   B. sanitizer
   C. fungicide
   D. sterilizer

208. Anything that destroys bacteria (applied especially to chemical agents that kill disease "germs," but not necessarily spores) is a
   A. sterilizer
   B. sanitizer
   C. germicide
   D. fungicide

209. The agent that reduces the bacteria count to "safe levels," as judged by public health requirements, is called a
   A. disinfectant
   B. fungicide
   C. germicide
   D. sanitizer

210. Anything that destroys yeast and mold is called a
    A. disinfectant
    B. fungicide
    C. germicide
    D. sanitizer

211. Bacteria come in which of the following shapes?
    1. Rod shapes
    2. Round or ball shapes
    3. Comma-shaped or spiral-shaped
    4. Square-shaped
        A. 1 and 2
        B. 1., 2., and 3
        C. 1., 2., and 4
        D. All of the above

212. Two bacillus bacteria connected together are called a
    A. *Streptobacillus*
    B. *Diplobacillus*
    C. *Vibrio*
    D. spirochete

213. Four rod-shaped bacteria connected together are called a
    A. *Streptobacillus*
    B. *Streptococcus*
    C. *Spirillum*
    D. *Staphylococcus*

214. Which of the following classifications of bacteria will live and grow in humans?
    A. Psychrophilic
    B. Mesophilic
    C. Thermophilic
    D. All of the above

215. Which of the following is NOT a chief characteristic of a virus?
  - **A.** Viruses cannot be seen with an ordinary light microscope
  - **B.** They are able to pass through filters that trap bacteria
  - **C.** They grow only on living tissue and cannot grow on culture media
  - **D.** They are true cells

216. Polio is caused by
  - **A.** Gram-negative bacteria
  - **B.** Gram-positive bacteria
  - **C.** virus
  - **D.** both A. and B.

217. What percentage of all patients admitted to general hospitals develops hospital-acquired pneumonia
  - **A.** 0.5% to 5.0%
  - **B.** 5% to 7.5%
  - **C.** 8% to 10%
  - **D.** 10% to 15%

218. Respiratory equipment has been isolated as the causative agent in the spread of which of the following?
  - **1.** *Pseudomonas*
  - **2.** *Flavobacterium*
  - **3.** *Herellea* species
  - **4.** *Alcaligenes*
    - **A.** 1. and 3.
    - **B.** 1. only
    - **C.** 2. and 4.
    - **D.** All of the above

219. Which of the following may be the initial sources of contamination from respiratory therapy equipment?
  - **A.** Contaminated medication
  - **B.** Contaminated water reservoirs
  - **C.** Contaminated nebulizer jets and venturi tubes
  - **D.** All of the above

220. Which of the following is a Gram-positive pathogen?
   1. *Klebsiella pneumoniae*
   2. *Pseudomonas aeruginosa*
   3. *Staphylococcus aureus*
   4. *Serratia marcescens*
      A. 1. and 2.
      B. 1. and 3.
      C. 3. only
      D. All of the above

221. *Mycobacterium tuberculosis* is a
   A. Gram-positive cocci pathogen
   B. Gram-positive rod pathogen
   C. Gram-positive spore-forming rod pathogen
   D. Gram-negative cocci pathogen

222. Which of the following pathogens is responsible for 80% of lobar pneumonia?
   A. *Streptococcus pneumoniae*
   B. *Klebsiella pneumoniae*
   C. *Escherichia coli*
   D. *Pseudomonas aeruginosa*

223. Which of the following are Gram-negative pathogens?
   1. *Pseudomonas aeruginosa*
   2. *Streptococcus pyogenes*
   3. *Klebsiella pneumoniae*
   4. *Streptococcus pneumoniae*
      A. 2. and 4.
      B. 1. and 3.
      C. 1., 2., and 4.
      D. All of the above

224. Which of the following pathogens is responsible for whooping cough?
   A. *Neisseria meningitis*
   B. *Bordetella pertussis*
   C. *Clostricium nouyi*
   D. *Haemophilus influenzae*

225. Normal flora found in the nasopharynx include
1. *Staphylococcus epidemidis*
2. *Neisseria* sp
3. *Viridans streptococci*
4. *Borrelia vincentii*
   - **A.** 1. and 2.
   - **B.** 2. and 4.
   - **C.** 1., 2., and 3.
   - **D.** all of the above

226. Normal flora found in lower respiratory tract are
- **A.** *Actinomyces israelii*
- **B.** *Candida albicans*
- **C.** *Haemophilus*
- **D.** none of the above

227. *Pseudomonas eruginosa* has been observed to pass through filters of what micron size?
- **A.** 0.10 μm
- **B.** 0.20 μm
- **C.** 0.35 μm
- **D.** 0.45 μm

228. Which of the following is incorrect about *Legionella pneumophilia*?
- **A.** It causes legionellosis
- **B.** It is a rod-shaped pathogen
- **C.** It grows on "routine" culture plates
- **D.** The mortality rate of treated patients is 5% to 10%

229. *Legionella* can be found in which of the following?
1. Soil
2. Drinking water
3. Freshwater lakes
4. Water at 40°C
   - **A.** 2. and 3.
   - **B.** 2. only
   - **C.** 3. and 4.
   - **D.** All of the above

230. Hepatitis B is caused by
    A. spore
    B. bacteria
    C. virus
    D. fungus

231. The prevalence of serologic markers for HBV infections (a reliable measure of previous infection) in the general population is 3% to 5%. In contrast, the documented studies of anesthesia personnel are
    A. 2% to 4%
    B. 8% to 10%
    C. 19% to 22%
    D. 25% to 30%

232. Acquired immunodeficiency syndrome is caused by
    A. bacteria
    B. mold
    C. virus
    D. fungus

233. The AIDS virus is called
    A. human T-cell lymphotrophic virus type III (HTLV-III)
    B. lymphadinopathy-associated virus (LAV)
    C. human immunodeficiency virus (HIV)
    D. all of the above

234. AIDS is trasmitted by all of the following except
    A. sexually
    B. blood from contaminated needles
    C. casual contact
    D. blood transfusions

235. The following statements for sterilization and disinfection procedures for HIV are correct except
    A. contaminated instruments should undergo routine sterilization and disinfection after use
    B. devices that contact intact mucus membranes should be sterilized or receive high-level disinfection
    C. germicides are not effective against HIV virus
    D. the usual sterilization procedures currently in use are effective

236. *Escherichia coli* is responsible for what percentage of hospital-acquired infections?
A. 10%
B. 25%
C. 45%
D. 65%

237. Which of the following is almost always responsible for the spread of nosocomial infection?
A. Food
B. People
C. Flies
D. None of the above

238. Microorganisms are transmitted by
1. coughing
2. sneezing
3. talking
4. yawning
A. 1. and 2.
B. 2. only
C. all of the above
D. none of the above

239. An uncovered sneeze can throw droplets of moisture as far away as
A. 2 ft
B. 5 ft
C. 10 ft
D. 15 ft

240. Direct transmission of microorganisms may be accomplished by
A. touch
B. sneeze
C. cough
D. all of the above

241. Indirect transmission of microorganisms may be accomplished by
    A. stethoscope
    B. money
    C. clothing
    D. all of the above

242. Which of the following generally has not been found to be a cause of nosocomial infection?
    A. Trained medical people
    B. Small volume medication nebulizer
    C. Food
    D. Ultrasonic nebulizers

243. The easiest and most often used method of preventing cross-infection is
    A. handwashing
    B. gown
    C. special rooms
    D. sterilization of equipment

244. Isolation procedures include
    A. special rooms
    B. special handwashing
    C. special material handling
    D. all of the above

245. Special isolation rooms usually require
    1. a closed door to stop the spread of particles from leaving the room
    2. ultraviolet lighting
    3. special ventilation to filter bacteria out of the hospital air-circulation system
    4. special air systems built in over, under, or around the patient's bed
    A. 1. and 2.
    B. 1. only
    C. 1., 3., and 4.
    D. all of the above

246. The body's first line of defense against microorganisms is
A. leukocyte
B. skin
C. antibiotic
D. mucosa

247. The principal factors that influence the ability to kill bacteria and other microorganisms are
1. strength of the killing agent
2. time the agent has to act
3. type of microorganism being killed
4. temperature of the environment
5. number of microbes to be killed
   A. 1., 2., and 3.
   B. 1., 2., and 4.
   C. 1. and 4.
   D. all of the above

248. A method for testing the killing power of some components and agents is called
A. Rideal Coefficient Test
B. Phenol Coefficient Test
C. Walker Coefficient Test
D. Bufalini Coefficient Test

249. Which of the following chemical agents has the strongest killing power?
A. An agent with a P.C. of 1
B. An agent with a P.C. of 3
C. An agent with a P.C. of 4
D. An agent with a P.C. of 5

250. When using steam autoclave procedures, which factors are most important for effectiveness?
1. Temperature
2. Time
3. Pressure
4. Type of microorganism
   A. 1. and 2.
   B. 1. and 3.
   C. 1. and 4.
   D. All of the above

251. What pressure is required for steam autoclave?
    A. 5 psi
    B. 10 psi
    C. 15 psi
    D. Pressure not required

252. The temperature of steam autoclave procedure is
    A. 80°C
    B. 100°C
    C. 120°C
    D. 140°C

253. Which of the following is incorrect about steam autoclave procedure?
    A. Does not kill spores
    B. Leaves no toxic residue
    C. Simple quality control
    D. Quick procedure

254. Which of the following are less desirable points of steam autoclave?
    1. Expensive to purchase and install
    2. Cannot be used on all equipment
    3. Can be dangerous
    4. Time-consuming procedure
        A. 2. and 3.
        B. 1., 2., and 3.
        C. 2. and 4.
        D. All of the above

255. Sterilization by pasteurization cannot be guaranteed because
    A. water temperatures vary
    B. materials must be dried and handled after procedure
    C. equipment must be loaded correctly
    D. water contains microorganisms which contaminate equipment

256. Cidex is
  A. used in gas sterilization
  B. activated glutaraldehyde
  C. used in pasteurization
  D. none of the above

257. Advantages of Cidex are
  1. easy to use
  2. kills all pathogens
  3. minimum corrosion
  4. sterilization is guaranteed
    A. 1. and 2.
    B. 1., 2., and 3.
    C. 1., 2., and 4.
    D. all of the above

258. Which of the following is not true when using ethylene oxide (toxic gas)?
  A. Kills all pathogens
  B. Simple quality control
  C. Long shelf life
  D. Quick procedure

259. Which of the following methods of sterilization does not kill spores?
  A. Steam autoclave
  B. Pasteurization
  C. Activated glutaraldehyde
  D. Ethylene oxide

260. Which of the following is not true of disposable equipment?
  A. All disposable equipment is packaged sterile
  B. It ensures quality control
  C. It makes efficient use of respiratory therapy personnel time
  D. it provides prepackaged, easy-to-use systems

261. The shelf life of gas-sterilized items wrapped in plastic wrap (heat sealed) is
    A. 15 to 30 days
    B. 30 to 60 days
    C. 90 to 100 days
    D. one year

262. The shelf life of gas-sterilized items wrapped in cloth is
    A. 15 to 30 days
    B. 30 to 60 days
    C. 90 to 100 days
    D. one year

263. Prior to sterilization, equipment should be
    A. washed clean of all organic matter
    B. rinsed completely
    C. air-dried
    D. all of the above

264. The shelf life of gas-sterilized items wrapped in plastic sealed with tape is
    A. 15 to 30 days
    B. 30 to 60 days
    C. 90 to 100 days
    D. one year

265. The normal percent of ethylene oxide that is used is
    A. 2% to 3%
    B. 5% to 8%
    C. 10% to 12%
    D. 15% to 20%

266. The effectiveness of ethylene oxide doubles for each _____ degree centigrade raise in temperature up to 60°C
    A. 5°C
    B. 10°C
    C. 15°C
    D. 20°C

Explanatory Answers

189. G. *Bacteria* are defined as microscopic, unicellular plants containing no chlorophyll. Reproduction occurs by binary fission. (**Ref.** 28, p. 237)

190. J. A cell capable of ingesting bacteria on any other foreign material is a *phagocyte.* (**Ref.** 28, p. 239)

191. A. When an organism is *aerobic* it is said to only be able to survive in a surrounding containing oxygen. (**Ref.** 28, p. 237)

192. C. A substance that prevents or arrests the growth or action of organisms by inhibiting their activity or destroying them is said to be an *antiseptic.* (**Ref.** 28, p. 237)

193. E. A device that is used to sterilize medical equipment by steam under pressure is called an *autoclave.* (**Ref.** 28, p. 237)

194. F. *Bacteremia* is a situation in which blood contains bacteria. This is not to imply that growth of bacteria occurs. (**Ref.** 28, p. 237)

195. I. A *pathogen* is a disease-producing microorganism or material. Any substance under the right circumstances may become pathogenic. (**Ref.** 28, p. 239)

196. B. *Anaerobic* refers to organisms that survive in atmosphere without oxygen. (**Ref.** 28, p. 237)

197. D. *Asepsis* refers to an environment that is completely free of all bacteria or microorganisms. (**Ref.** 28, p. 237)

198. H. *Commensalism* refers to a symbiotic (peaceful) association between two organisms without the harming of one another. (**Ref.** 28, p. 238)

199. D. *Flora, transient* refer to the surface bacteria which can be removed by handwashing. (**Ref.** 28, p. 238)

200. F. *Gram-negative organisms* appear red when stained with the technique known as Gram staining. (**Ref.** 28, p. 238)

201. A. Bacteria that appear as rods under a microscope are termed *bacilli.* (**Ref.** 28, p. 237)

202. G. Organisms that are slender, flexuous, or corkscrew-shaped and are highly mobile are termed *spirochetes.* (**Ref.** 28, p. 239)

203. C. Some bacteria cannot be removed by ordinary washing. They reside below the surface of the skin in pores, cracks, and folds of skin. They are called *flora, resident.* (**Ref.** 22, p. 238)

204. B. *Cocci* are bacteria shaped like dots, circles, or spheres under a microscope. (**Ref.** 28, p. 238)

205. F. Any organism that appears blue upon Gram stain is said to be *Gram-positive* (**Ref.** 28, p. 238)

206. A. *Sterilization* is the process that destroys all forms of life, including bacteria, mold, spores, and viruses. The process itself may be chemical or physical in nature. (**Ref.** 28, p. 239)

207. A. A *disinfectant* is a substance usually applied to inanimate objects for the purpose of destroying germs that cause diseases. Disinfectants, however, do not necessarily destroy resistant forms of spores. (**Ref.** 28, p. 238)

208. C. *Germicides* can also destroy bacteria and often are chemical agents; however they do not necessarily kill spores. (**Ref.** 28, p. 238)

209. D. Agents that reduce bacteria to what is termed safe levels by public health requirements are called *sanitizers.* (**Ref.** 28, p. 239)

210. B. *Fungicides* are anything that destroy fungi (yeasts and molds). They may be applied to living or inanimate objects. (**Ref.** 28, p. 238)

211. C. Bacteria are essentially three different shapes: rods, round- or ball-shaped, or spirals. Within each shape bacteria can also take many other forms, such as chains or clusters. (**Ref.** 28, p. 239)

212. B. Two bacilli that are connected are called *Diplobacillus*. A *Streptobacillus* refers to four rods joined in a chain. *Vibrio* belongs to spiral class of bacteria as does a spirochete. (**Ref.** 28, p. 240)

213. A. *Streptobacillus* is a chain of four rods. *Streptococcus* is a chain of round-shaped bacteria. *Staphylococcus* is a cluster of round-shaped bacteria, while *Spirillum* is a rigid spiral with one or more twists in its shape. (**Ref.** 28, p. 240)

214. B. Mesophilic bacteria survive in temperatures between 20° and 40°C, well within the normal body temperature. Psychrophilic bacteria live in environments of 0° to 25°C and thermophilic bacteria live in temperatures of 45° to 70°C. (**Ref.** 28, p. 241)

215. D. Viruses are not true cells. They act as parasites using cells to replicate their genetic material. They cannot be seen through an ordinary light microscope, are able to pass through bacteria filters, and only grow on living tissue. They cannot exist in culture media. (**Ref.** 28, p. 242)

216. C. Polio is caused by a virus. (**Ref.** 28, p. 242)

217. A. In 1970 the Centers for Disease Control reported that from 0.5% to 5% of all patients admitted to general hospitals developed hospital-acquired pneumonia. Respiratory equipment was noted as a prime causative agent. (**Ref.** 28, p. 243)

218. D. Nosocomial infections can be spread through respiratory equipment. Some of the bacteria named as pathogens from equipment include *Pseudomonas, Flavobacterium, Herellea* species, and *Alcaligenes.* (**Ref.** 28, p. 243)

219. D. Sources of potential colonization of bacteria may include medications that have been contaminated, water reservoirs, contaminated nebulizers, and venturi tubes. Contaminated aerosols that are deposited beyond ciliated bronchial tissue may result in colonization with eventual spreading to other areas of the lung. (**Ref.** 28, p. 243)

220. C. *Staphylococcus aureaus* is a Gram-positive organism that is part of the normal flora of the skin, mouth, and nasal mucous membranes. It can be responsible for food poisoning, septicemia, pneumonia, and abscesses. *Klebsiella, Pseudomonas,* and *Serratia* are all Gram-negative pathogens that are often opportunistic organisms. (**Ref.** 28, p. 245)

221. B. *Mycobacterium tuberculosis* is a Gram-positive pathogen (rod) which is the causative agent of tuberculosis. (**Ref.** 28, p. 244)

222. A. A Gram-positive cocci known as *Streptococcus pneumoniae* is responsible for 80% of lobar pneumonia. *E. coli* is more responsible for gastrointestinal infections and urinary tract infections. *Klebsiella* and *Serratia* are Gram-negative pathogens also associated with respiratory infections. (**Ref.** 28, p. 244)

223. B. *Pseudomonas* and *Klebsiella* are both Gram-negative rods responsible for pulmonary infections. *Streptococcus pyogenes* are responsible for "strep throat," fever, and tonsillitis. *Streptococcus pneumoniae* is responsible for 80% of all lobar pneumonias. (**Ref.** 28, p. 244)

224. B. Whooping cough is caused by a Gram-negative rod called *Bordetalla pertussis. Neisseria meningitis* causes meningococcal meningitis, while *Clostricium nouyi* is responsible for gas gangrene. *Haemophilus influenzae,* once thought to be the "flu," is now associated with a fatal infant form of meningitis. (**Ref.** 28, p. 244)

225. C. The nasopharynx is colonized by bacteria that include *Neisseria, Staphylococcus epidermidis,* and *viridans streptococci.* Under certain conditions these organisms may invade the lower respiratory tract and become pathogenic. (**Ref.** 36, p. 84)

226. D. The sterility of the lower respiratory tract is maintained by many protective mechanisms, including the ciliary tree, mucous blanket, cough, macrophages, and sneeze. (**Ref.** 36, p. 84)

227. D. Although *Pseudomonas* generally has a mass size of 0.50 μ, it has been observed to pass through filters of 0.45 μ. (**Ref.** 36, p. 85)

228. C. Legionellosis is an acute human infection caused by *Legionella pneumophilia.* It is a rod-shaped pathogen that can only be cultured on special media culture. Its mortality rate, if untreated, is 15% to 20%, but when treated falls to 5% to 10%. (**Ref.** 37, p. 4)

229. D. *Legionella* has been found in soil which may become airborne during excavation. It has been discovered in freshwater lakes and drinking water, but interestingly enough, direct ingestion has not been shown to cause legionellosis. The bacteria flourish between 32° and 40°C with the highest incidence of outbreak between June and November. (**Ref.** 37, p. 4)

230. C. Hepatitis B is caused by a virus which is transmitted from host to host via blood or body fluids. It is treatable, but may go on to be chronic in 10% of those infected. Symptoms may be minimal or life-threatening. (**Ref.** 38, p. 84)

231. C. All hospital workers at risk for blood or body fluid exposure have an increased seropositivity to hepatitis B virus. Documented studies of anesthesia personnel have shown a 19% to 22% prevalence. (**Ref.** 38, p. 84)

232. C. Acquired immunodeficiency syndrome was discovered in 1984 by two separate groups. It is caused by a retrovirus containing RNA that is transcribed in reverse to the host cells' DNA. (**Ref.** 38, p. 86)

233. D. The AIDS virus has been labeled by many names, including human T-cell lymphotrophic virus type three (HtLV-III); lymphadinopathy-associated virus (LAV); or by its most common name, human immunodeficiency virus (HIV). (**Ref.** 38, p. 86)

234. C. AIDS has only been proven to spread by exchange of blood or body fluids. This occurs either by contaminated needles or unsafe sex. Blood transfusions have been reported as a cause; however, universal testing now occurs on all blood donors. HIV can also be transmitted perinatally. Casual contact has not been shown to promote transmission. (**Ref.** 38, p. 85)

235. C. Routine sterilization procedures currently practiced are effective against the AIDS virus. Instruments or devices that come in contact with infected material should be sterilized or disinfected. Germicides should be used on surfaces exposed to blood or body fluids. It should be stressed that these practices should be used in the care of all patients, as incubation periods do not allow for complete knowledge of one's possible diseases. (**Ref.** 38, p. 85)

236. C. *Escherichia coli* is a bacteria that is part of the gastrointestinal normal flora. It can be responsible for pathogenic diseases such as pneumonia, endocarditis, meningitis, and urinary tract infections. It accounts for 45% of all nosocomial infections. (**Ref.** 22, p. 573)

237. B. The spread of disease usually occurs by four mechanisms: fingers, flies, families, and food; however, people are almost always at fault for the transmission of nosocomial infections. (**Ref.** 28, p. 246)

238. C. Microbes can be spread by coughing, sneezing, talking, and yawning. Particles can remain suspended in the atmosphere for hours after being coughed or sneezed out. (**Ref.** 28, p. 246)

239. C. Particles from an uncovered sneeze can travel as far as 10 ft. This can also be demonstrated from exhaled particles from an intermittant positive pressure breathing circuit. (**Ref.** 28, p. 246)

240. D. In direct transmission of microbes, physical contact is not necessary. Transmission can occur from touching, coughing, or sneezing. (**Ref.** 28, p. 246)

241. D. Indirect transmission occurs when transmission occurs from host to host through some other mediator. These include food, water, money, clothing, dust, or even an unclean stethoscope. (**Ref.** 28, p. 246)

242. B. Small volume medication nebulizers, so long as they are properly cleaned and not used patient-to-patient, have not been found to be a cause of nosocomial infections. (**Ref.** 228, p. 247)

243. A. Handwashing is the easiest and most often used method to prevent the transmission of infection. It is cost-effective and no special equipment is required to facilitate its use. (**Ref.** 28, p. 247)

244. D. Isolation procedures include the use of special rooms to prevent bacteria from either entering or leaving a room, special handwashing using bacteriostatic soap to aid in the removal of bacteria, and special material handling to assure the proper disposal of contaminated material. (**Ref.** 28, p. 247)

245. C. Isolation rooms should possess attributes which include a self-closing door to prevent bacteria from entering or leaving a room; special ventilation to filter bacteria present in the atmosphere; and special air systems built over, under, or around the patient's bed. (**Ref.** 28, p. 247)

246. B. The body's skin is the first line of defense against infection. It is essentially impervious to water, oil and dirt, and microbes so long as there is no cut or break. (**Ref.** 28, p. 247)

247. D. There are six factors that influence the ability of certain agents to kill microbes. These include the strength of solution used, the time that the agent is exposed to the bacteria, the temperature the bacteria are exposed to (if increased it will decrease the time necessary to kill bacteria), the type of bacteria being killed (spores are most resistant), and finally the number of microbes and the environment they exist in. (**Ref.** 28, p. 248)

248. B. In 1903 Rideal and Walker developed a test known as the Plenol Coefficient (P.C.) to measure the killing power of certain agents as compared to phenol. However, this test is of little use in evaluating nonphenol-type compounds. (**Ref.** 28, p. 249)

249. D. Phenol coefficient refers to how strong a substance is in relation to the killing strength of phenol. (**Ref.** 28, p. 249)

250. D. When autoclaving is the sterilization method of choice, temperature (120°C), pressure (15 psi), and time (dependent on type of material) all play critical roles in its effectiveness. Another variability is the type of microbe; spores require longer autoclave exposure than do other microbes. (**Ref.** 28, p. 250)

251. C. When autoclaving, a pressure of 15 psi is required. Of note: pressure alone or temperature alone does not assure full sterility. (**Ref.** 28, p. 250)

252. C. The temperature required during steam autoclaving is 120°C along with a 15 psi pressure source. (**Ref.** 28, p. 250)

253. A. Steam autoclaving kills all pathogens, including spores. It is relatively quick and uses no toxic materials. It allows the material being autoclaved to be wrapped prior to the procedure, which maintains sterility following the procedure. (**Ref.** 28, p. 250)

254. B. Disadvantages of steam autoclaving include the fact that all equipment cannot be autoclaved, it is an expensive system to install, and there is some degree of danger with the amount of pressure and temperature levels used. (**Ref.** 28, p. 250)

255. B. Although pasteurization can produce sterilization, the processing requires that the material must be dried and handled following the procedure. Therefore, contamination may occur. Generally water temperature remains stable at 60°C which will kill all microbes except spores when equipment is loaded correctly. (**Ref.** 28, p. 250)

256. B. Cidex is the brand name for activated glutaraldehyde. It is available in liquid form which is used to soak contaminated material. It only requires 15 min, but is generally limited to smaller pieces of equipment. (**Ref.** 28, p. 250)

257. B. Although Cidex is easy to use, results in minimal corrosion, and kills all pathogens, including spores when used properly, sterilization is not guaranteed because, like pasturization, this process requires handling following treatment. (**Ref.** 28, p. 250)

258. D. Use of ethylene oxide will guarantee sterility because the material is packaged prior to treatment. The excellent quality control measures ensure long shelf life no matter how large the equipment is. Some disadvantages include high cost, use of toxic gas, and the requirement of a (aeration) procedure which may last up to seven days in some circumstances. (**Ref.** 28, p. 250)

259. B. When properly used, autoclaving, Cidex, or ethylene oxide will guarantee sterilization. Pasturization will kill all pathogens except spores. (**Ref.** 28, p. 250)

260. A. Disposable equipment is easy to use and ensures quality control because sterilization procedures are eliminated. With the elimination of processing, personnel time can be more efficiently used. Its disadvantages include cost and the amount of storage space required. (**Ref.** 28, p. 251)

261. D. Material wrapped in plastic which was heat sealed and exposed to ethylene oxide will remain sterile for up to one year. (**Ref.** 28, p. 252)

262. A. Any material wrapped in cloth and exposed to ethylene oxide will possess a shelf life of 15 to 30 days. Material in plastic sealed with tape will remain sterile for 90 to 100 days. (**Ref.** 28, p. 252)

263. D. Prior to sterilization all equipment must be washed and cleaned of any organic matter. They must then be rinsed thoroughly and allowed to air dry. (**Ref.** 22, p. 280)

264. C. Items wrapped in plastic sealed with tape which is exposed to ethylene oxide will remain sterile for 90 to 100 days. Cloth wrap will have a shelf life of 15 to 30 days while paper wrap will last 30 to 60 days. Only heat sealed plastic will remain sterile for up to one year. (**Ref.** 28, p. 252)

265. C. Ethylene oxide is usually combined with either carbon dioxide or Freon in a 10% to 12% mixture that is nonflammable as long as the temperature remains below 55°C. Higher mixtures are dangerous due to their flammability. (**Ref.** 22, p. 583)

266. B. For every 10°C rise in temperature, the effectiveness of ethylene oxide doubles, up to a temperature of 60°C. Typical systems run at a temperature of 54°C, thereby limiting the danger of explosion. (**Ref.** 22, p. 583)

7 Medical Gas Production, Storage, and Control

DIRECTIONS (Questions 267–277): Each of the questions or incomplete statements below is followed by four suggested answers or completions. Select the **one** that is **best** in each case.

---

267. The agency that regulates shipping, filling, marking, and labeling of gas cylinders is
    A. Department of Transportation (DOT)
    B. Bureau of Medical Devices
    C. Compressed Gas Association (CGA)
    D. Department of Health and Human Services (HHS)

268. Which agency regulates handling and storage of cylinders, piping, fittings, and cylinder markings?
    A. National Fire Protection Association (NFPA)
    B. CGA
    C. HHS
    D. American Standards Association

269. Which agency regulates the standards for all medical devices and classification of medical devices?
    A. International Standards Organization (ISO)
    B. CGA
    C. Bureau of Medical Devices
    D. DOT

270. The Pin Index Safety System was originally described by
    A. American Standard System
    B. NFPA
    C. CGA
    D. HHS

271. The Pin Index Safety System is used
    A. to prevent inadvertent connection of the wrong gas, in a small cylinder (A,B,D,E) to all medical gas dispensing equipment
    B. to prevent inadvertent administration of the wrong gas from a central piping system
    C. only with anesthesia equipment
    D. all of the above

272. The Pin Index Safety System provides for a variety of combinations, each using two position holes in the cylinder valve to correspond with pins in the yoke. How many combinations are there?
    A. 6
    B. 8
    C. 10
    D. 12

273. The PISS position for oxygen is
    A. 2 to 6
    B. 2 to 5
    C. 3 to 5
    D. 1 to 5

274. The PISS position for compressed air is
    A. 2 to 5
    B. 3 to 5
    C. 1 to 5
    D. 4 to 6

275. The PISS position for nitrous oxide is
    A. 2 to 5
    B. 3 to 5
    C. 4 to 6
    D. 2 to 6

276. Cylinders are tested every
    1. 3 years
    2. 5 years
    3. 7 years
    4. 10 years
        A. 1. only
        B. 1. and 2.
        C. 2. and 4.
        D. 2. only

277. Small cylinders use a fusable plug designed to melt at a temperature of
    A. 100 to 110°F
    B. 120 to 140°F
    C. 150 to 170°F
    D. 190 to 200°F

DIRECTIONS (Questions 278–288): Each group of questions below consists of a set of lettered words or phrases, followed by a list of numbered items. For each lettered word or phrase, select the correct numbered item. Each lettered word or phrase may be used more than once or not at all.

Questions 278–282: Select the correct lettered description for each numbered gas or gas mixture.

    A. Combustible
    B. Supports combustion
    C. Inert

278. Oxygen

279. Helium

280. Carbon dioxide

281. Carbon dioxide and oxygen

282. Helium and oxygen

Questions 283-288: Select the correct lettered color code for each numbered gas or gas mixture.

    A. Gray
    B. Black
    C. Blue
    D. Varies by manufacturer
    E. Light green body; gray shoulder
    F. Light green
    G. Brown

283. Oxygen

284. Nitrous oxide

285. Nitrogen

286. Helium

287. Carbon dioxide

288. Carbon dioxide and oxygen mixture

Explanatory Answers

267. A. The Department of Transportation (DOT) is responsible for all regulations pertaining to the shipping, filling, marking, and labeling of gas cylinders. On each cylinder you should see DOT imprinted near the neck of the cylinder. (**Ref.** 28, p. 122)

268. B. The Compressed Gas Association (CGA) is the regulatory body responsible for the storage and handling of cylinder markings. The National Fire Protection Association develops the standards regarding storage and delivery which the CGA follows. The Department of Health and Human Services (HHS) regulates the quality and purity of medical gas while the American Standards Association is responsible for the prevention of inadvertent gas delivery through the use of gas-specific regulators. (**Ref.** 28, p. 122)

269. C. The Bureau of Medical Devices regulates the standards and classifications for all medical devices. The Compressed Gas Association is for the storage and handling of medical gas, while the Department of Transportation regulates the shipping and marking of cylinders. The International Standards Organization is an international body responsible for the standardization of medical equipment, fittings, and for terminology and testing. (**Ref.** 28, p. 122)

270. B. The Pin Index Safety System was originally developed by the NFPA in 1952 for the prevention of inadvertent attachment of a gas-specific regulating device to an inappropriate gas cylinder. (**Ref.** 28, p. 123)

271. A. To prevent inadvertent attachment of a gas-specific regulator to the incorrect medical gas, the Pin Index Safety System was developed. To prevent inadvertent gas administration of a wrong gas from a central piping line the diameter index safety system was developed. It can be used anywhere small cylinders are utilized. (A,B,D,E sizes) (**Ref.** 39)

272. C. Although the Pin Index Safety System only has 6 pin fittings, using combinations of two holes allows for 10 possible individual combinations. (**Ref.** 39)

273. B. The Pin Index Safety System utilizes the positions of 2 and 5 for oxygen. (**Ref.** 28, p. 123)

274. C. The Pin Index Safety System uses positions 1 and 5 for compressed air. (**Ref.** 28, p. 120)

275. B. Nitrous oxide cylinders use PISS positions 3 and 5. Helium–oxygen mixtures are 4–6 while carbon dioxide uses 2 and 6. (**Ref.** 28, p. 123)

276. C. Cylinders are required to be tested every 5 years unless they are marked by a star next to the test date. This indicates a 10-year cycle. (**Ref.** 28, p. 125)

277. C. Small cylinders have a fuseable plug located at the stem which is designed to melt at a temperature of 150 to 170°F. (**Ref.** 22, p. 361)

278. B. Oxygen is a potential hazard if not handled properly. Although by itself it will not burn, objects exposed to oxygen will burn more rapidly. (**Ref.** 28, p. 120)

279. C. Helium is a colorless, odorless gas which is inert and nonexplosive. Its primary medical use is for partial airway obstructions. (**Ref.** 28, p. 120)

280. C. Carbon dioxide alone is inert and is noncombustible. In fact, it is primarily used for the elimination of combustion. (**Ref.** 28, p. 120)

281. B. Carbon dioxide mixed with oxygen will also only support combustion, although to a lesser degree than oxygen alone. Its primary medical use is to increase respirations and to dilate cerebral blood vessels. (**Ref.** 28, p. 120)

282. B. Helium–oxygen mixtures will only support combustion and are generally used for the treatment of partial airway obstructions. (**Ref.** 28, p. 120)

283. F. Oxygen is stored in light green cylinders within the

United States. Some foreign countries utilize the color white. (**Ref.** 22, p. 361)

284. C. Nitrous oxide is maintained in blue cylinders. (**Ref.** 22, p. 361)

285. B. A black cylinder would indicate that the contents consist of nitrogen. (**Ref.** 22, p. 361)

286. G. Helium would be stored in a brown cylinder. (**Ref.** 22, p. 361)

287. A. Carbon dioxide is stored in gray cylinders. (**Ref.** 22, p. 361)

288. E. Carbon dioxide–oxygen mixtures are required to be stored in green cylinders with the top portion painted gray. (**Ref.** 22, p. 361)

8 Equipment and Procedures

DIRECTIONS (Questions 289–315): Each of the questions or incomplete statements below is followed by four suggested answers or completions. Select the **one** that is **best** in each case.

289. The capacity of an oxygen E-cylinder is
    A. 12.7 ft^2
    B. 22 ft^2
    C. 28 ft^2
    D. 32 ft^2

290. An H-cylinder of oxygen has a capacity of
    A. 187 ft^2
    B. 200 ft^2
    C. 244 ft^2
    D. 276 ft^2

291. The maximum filling pressure of an oxygen cylinder is
    A. 500 psi
    B. 1500 psi
    C. 2200 psi
    D. varies with cylinder size

292. A G-cylinder has a capacity of 187 ft². What is the factor for duration of flow?
   A. .005
   B. 2.41
   C. 3.14
   D. 6.61

293. A patient is being transported with an oxygen E-cylinder with a gauge pressure of 1500 psi at a liter flow of 4 L/min. When will the cylinder run empty?
   A. 1 hr and 45 min
   B. 1 hr and 15 min
   C. 55 min
   D. 45 min

294. A patient at home is using an H-cylinder to administer oxygen via a 6 L/min nasal cannula. The cylinder gauge pressure is 1400 psi and the patient changes the cylinder when 200 psi is remaining. How long does the patient have to wait before changing the cylinder?
   A. 10.5 hr
   B. 12.2 hr
   C. 20 hr
   D. None of the above

295. High-pressure gas regulators reduce cylinder pressures to a working pressure of
   A. 200 psi
   B. 100 psi
   C. 50 psi
   D. 25 psi

296. A high pressure pop-off valve is incorporated into a single-step regulator. At what pressure is this valve set?
   A. 100 psi
   B. 150 psi
   C. 200 psi
   D. 250 psi

297. Which type of flowmeter will indicate a flow higher than actual flow if back pressure is applied distal to the gauge?
A. Bourdon
B. Thorpe
C. Compensated Thorpe
D. Uncompensated Thorpe

298. Which type of flowmeter will indicate a flow lower than actual flow if back pressure is applied distal to the needle valve?
A. Bourdon
B. Thorpe
C. Compensated Thorpe
D. Uncompensated Thorpe

299. Which type of flowmeter will indicate the actual flow if back pressure is applied distal to the needle valve?
A. Bourdon
B. Thorpe
C. Compensated Thorpe
D. Uncompensated Thorpe

300. Flowmeters are calculated to operate at which pressure?
A. 35 to 65 psig
B. 45 to 55 psig
C. 35 to 50 psig
D. 45 to 65 psig

301. Which of the following factors determine the accuracy of Thorpe tube flowmeters
A. position
B. inlet gas pressure
C. faulty valve seat
D. all of the above

302. A Bourdon-type flowmeter is most accurate with a flow rate of
A. 1 to 3 L/min
B. 3 to 7 L/min
C. 8 to 10 L/min
D. greater than 10 L/min

303. Oxygen delivery systems are divided into which categories?
1. Low-flow systems
2. Demand systems
3. Closed systems
4. High-flow systems
    A. 1. and 4.
    B. 1., 2., and 4.
    C. 2. and 3.
    D. All of the above

304. The FIO_2 delivered with any low-flow system is
1. extremely accurate
2. extremely variable
3. measurable
4. unpredictable
    A. 1. and 3.
    B. 2. only
    C. 2. and 4.
    D. 2. and 3.

305. If the patient's minute volume were to increase on a particular low-flow system, the FIO_2 would
A. increase
B. decrease
C. remain the same
D. only be affected by change in liter flow

306. If a patient were on a 4 L nasal cannula with a tidal volume of 500 and a respiratory rate of 20 breaths/min, his or her estimated FIO_2 delivered would be
1. I:E ratio: 1:2
2. inspiratory time: 1 sec
3. volume of patient's anatomical reservoir: 60 cc
    A. 0.30 FIO_2
    B. 0.36 FIO_2
    C. 0.39 FIO_2
    D. 0.43 FIO_2

307. A simple oxygen mask should be run at what liter flow?
  A. 3 to 5 L/min
  B. 5 to 8 L/min
  C. 8 to 10 L/min
  D. 10 to 12 L/min

308. Running a simple mask at the appropriate liter flow will result in an FIO_2 between
  A. 0.30 and 0.50
  B. 0.40 and 0.60
  C. 0.50 and 0.70
  D. none of the above

309. A partial rebreathing mask should be run at a liter flow
  A. to ensure that the bag deflates the whole way during inspiration
  B. to ensure that the bag deflates only about one-third during inspiration
  C. to ensure that the bag deflates about two-thirds during inspiration
  D. to prevent the bag from collapsing during inspiration

310. The partial rebreathing mask delivers an FIO_2 between
  A. 0.40 and 0.60
  B. 0.50 and 0.70
  C. 0.70 and 0.80+
  D. none of the above

311. A nonrebreathing mask should be run at a liter flow of
  A. 3 to 5 L/min
  B. 5 to 8 L/min
  C. 8 to 10 L/min
  D. 10 to 12 L/min

312. Running a nasal cannula at flow rates higher than 6 L/min will
  A. increase FIO_2 above 0.50
  B. cause oxygen toxicity
  C. irritate the mucosa
  D. benefit patient

313. Nasal cannulas need not be humidified if run at liter flows of
   A. 6 L/min or less
   B. 5 L/min or less
   C. 4 L/min or less
   D. none of the above

314. All of the following are true about nasal cannula oxygen therapy except
   A. FIO_2 may exceed 0.50
   B. can cause patients with COPD to stop breathing, resulting in death from asphyxia
   C. should not be used with patients who breathe through their mouths
   D. can present a fire hazard

315. A venturi-type mask can be in error by
   A. ±2%
   B. ±4%
   C. ±6%
   D. ±8%

DIRECTIONS (Questions 316–319): The group of questions below consists of a set of lettered items, followed by a list of numbered items. For each lettered item, select the correct numbered item.

Questions 316–319: Select the typical oxygen-to-air entrainment ratio for oxygen percentage for venturi-type mask.

   A. 3:1
   B. 10:1
   C. 20:1
   D. 5:1

316. 24%

317. 28%

318. 35%

319. 40%

DIRECTIONS (Questions 320–351): Each of the questions or incomplete statements below is followed by four suggested answers or completions. Select the **one** that is **best** in each case.

---

320. Nasal oxygen catheters should be alternated between nostrils every
   A. 4 to 8 hr
   B. 12 to 24 hr
   C. 24 to 36 hr
   D. 36 to 48 hr

321. Which of the following provides little advantage over a oxygen cannula or catheter?
   A. Nonrebreathing mask
   B. Simple mask
   C. Partial rebreathing mask
   D. Air-entrainment mask (venturi-type mask)

322. Most bubble humidifiers increase the relative humidity of oxygen from zero at ambient temperature to
   A. 60% to 70%
   B. 70% to 80%
   C. 80% to 90%
   D. 90% to 95%

323. A humidity deficit occurs between the inspired air and respiratory mucosa when the water content of inspired gas is less than:
   A. 43.8 mg/L at 37°C
   B. 40.8 mg/L at 37°C
   C. 38.5 mg/L at 37°C
   D. 34.3 mg/L at 37°C

324. Humidity deficit results in
   A. mucosal dehydration
   B. increased viscosity of the mucus
   C. decreased mucociliary clearance
   D. all of the above

325. Unheated bubble humidifiers provide what percentage of relative humidity at body temperature?
   A. 100%
   B. 60% to 70%
   C. 45% to 55%
   D. 30% to 40%

326. The approximate distance that a nasal catheter is to be inserted can be estimated by
   A. measuring the distance from the tragus of the ear to the tip of the nose.
   B. inserting the catheter until seen in oropharynx and pulling back 1 in.
   C. inserting 3 to 4 in.
   D. asking the patient if he or she is comfortable

327. The particle size range of ultrasonic nebulizers is
   A. 1 to 5 μ
   B. 3 to 8 μ
   C. 1 to 10 μ
   D. 8 to 15 μ

328. The average micron size overall for an ultrasonic nebulizer is
   A. 3 μ
   B. 5 μ
   C. 8 μ
   D. 10 μ

329. Because of inherent jet restriction, the maximum oxygen flow rate that can power most large-reservoir nebulizers is
   A. 10 to 12 L/min at 50 psi
   B. 12 to 14 L/min at 50 psi
   C. 14 to 16 L/min at 50 psi
   D. 16 to 18 L/min at 50 psi

330. Ultrasonic nebulizers break up solutions into particles using
    A. jet stream
    B. heat
    C. sound waves
    D. baffles

331. A mechanical nebulizer has an output of up to
    A. 1 to 1.5 mL/min
    B. 5 mL/min
    C. 8 mL/min
    D. 10 mL/min

332. A Babington nebulizer has an output of up to
    A. 3 mL/min
    B. 6 mL/min
    C. 8 mL/min
    D. 10 mL/min

333. Which of the following nebulizers produces the highest percentage of particles between 1 and 5 μm?
    A. Bird 500 mL nebulizer
    B. Puritan Bennett all-purpose nebulizer
    C. Ultrasonic nebulizer
    D. Babington nebulizer

334. Which of the following nebulizers has a small hollow glass sphere?
    A. Mechanical nebulizer
    B. Ultrasonic nebulizer
    C. Babington nebulizer
    D. A. and C.

335. Which of the following ventilators incorporates fluidic logic?
    A. Monaghan 225
    B. Sechrist IV-100B
    C. Ohio 550
    D. All of the above

336. The basic phenomenon responsible for overall fluidic mechanism is
A. Coanda effect
B. Bistable effect
C. Effie effect
D. Asymmetric effect

337. In a fluidic system, changes in direction of flow are accomplished by
A. backpressure
B. subatmospheric pressure
C. amplification
D. all of the above

338. Which of the following is not correct about endotracheal tube suctioning?
A. Should only be performed when indicated
B. Should be performed routinely or prophylactically
C. The catheter may traumatize respiratory tract mucosa
D. It predisposes to significant hypoxemia

339. Complications of traumatized respiratory tract mucosa include
A. mucosal erosion and hemorrhage
B. increased incidence of bacterial colonization
C. depression of the mucociliary clearance mechanism
D. all of the above

340. When performing tracheal suctioning, suction should be applied for
A. less than 15 sec
B. 15 to 30 sec
C. 20 to 40 sec
D. 30 to 45 sec

341. Hyperoxygenation ($FIO_2 = 1:0$) with manual inflation should be performed
A. prior to suctioning
B. after suctioning
C. both A. and B.
D. not at all because of hypoxic drive

342. When selecting a suction catheter
   A. the length of the catheter should be at least 18 in.
   B. the catheter diameter should be equal to or less than one-half the internal diameter of the airway
   C. it should be transparent
   D. all of the above

343. Which of the following are indications for the administration of IPPB?
   1. To improve delivery of medications in patients who are unable to coordinate their breathing patterns
   2. To improve coughing and expectoration
   3. To decrease a raising $PaCO_2$
   4. To decrease pulmonary distress
      A. 1. only
      B. 1. and 2.
      C. 1. and 3.
      D. All of the above

344. When administering IPPB, the measured IPPB tidal volume should
   A. equal spontaneous tidal volume
   B. equal maximum inspired volume
   C. Exceed spontaneous tidal volume by more than 25%
   D. it is not necessary to measure IPPB tidal volumes

345. IPPB may be unnecessary postoperatively if postoperative inspiratory capacity (IC) is within what percent of preoperative IC?
   A. 40% to 50%
   B. 30% to 40%
   C. 10% to 20%
   D. 5% to 10%

346. Important aspects of sustained maximal inspiration (SMI) are
1. the inspired volume
2. the device used
3. duration of end-inspiratory hold
4. preoperative baseline
  A. 1. and 2.
  B. 1. and 3.
  C. 1. and 4.
  D. all of the above

347. If it is necessary to deflate the cuff of a tracheostomy, what safeguard must be taken?
  A. Trachea must be suctioned
  B. Area above the cuff should be suctioned as well as possible through the pharynx
  C. Immediate tracheal suctioning following deflation
  D. All of the above

348. When are the best sputum culture specimens from a tracheostomy obtained?
  A. After trach care is performed
  B. After rinsing catheter with normal saline solution
  C. After postural drainage is maneuvered
  D. All of the above

349. Which of the following steps are incorrect for suctioning technique?
  A. Insert catheter with vacuum until it is obviously past the tip of the airway and approximately at the level of the carina
  B. Leave the suction catheter in airway for 30 sec
  C. Give 100% O_2 prior to and after suctioning
  D. A. and B.

350. The ideal suction catheter would
  A. have side holes
  B. be 20 to 22 in. long
  C. smooth molded ends
  D. all of the above

351. Which of the following complications are caused by airway suctioning?
   A. Lung collapse
   B. Hypotension
   C. Arrhythmia
   D. All of the above

Mechanical Ventilator Terminology and Classification

DIRECTIONS (Questions 352–360): Each group of questions below consists of a set of lettered items, followed by a list of numbered words or phrases. For each lettered item, select the correct numbered word or phrase.

Questions 352–356: For each lettered item, select the correct numbered definition.

   A. Positive pressure ventilator
   B. Negative pressure ventilator
   C. Powering mechanism
   D. Driving mechanism
   E. Limit

352. Provides the mechanical force that produces the flow of gas necessary for delivery of tidal volumes.

353. Makes use of a subatmospheric pressure applied to the thorax to deliver tidal volumes.

354. A physical parameter that cannot be exceeded, but is not the primary cycling mechanism.

355. Makes use of a supra-atmospheric pressure applied to the airway to deliver tidal volumes.

356. Physical energy source that provides the power for ventilator function.

Questions 357–360: For each lettered gas flow pattern, select the correct numbered pressure pattern.

- **A.** Square wave
- **B.** Decelerating flow
- **C.** Sine wave
- **D.** Accelerating flow

357. Sigmoidal

358. Nonlinear

359. Rectilinear

360. Parabalic

DIRECTIONS (Questions 361–372): Each of the questions or incomplete statements below is followed by four suggested answers or completions. Select the **one** that is **best** in each case.

---

361. Which of the following are available powering mechanisms?
- **A.** Electric
- **B.** Pneumatic
- **C.** Combined electric/pneumatic
- **D.** All of the above

362. The ability of a ventilator to maintain a consistent gas flow pattern is dependent on
1. the driving mechanism of the ventilator
2. the power mechanism of the ventilator
3. the total patient resistance to ventilation
4. the number of circuits
   - **A.** 1. only
   - **B.** 2. and 3.
   - **C.** 1. and 3.
   - **D.** 2. and 4.

363. A ventilator is considered a flow generator if the maximum pressure generated by the driving force is at least how many times the highest system pressure developed during gas delivery?
  A. 2
  B. 3
  C. 5
  D. 8

364. A ventilator that does meet the criteria as stated above is
  A. volume generator
  B. pressure generator
  C. flow generator
  D. time generator

365. Which of the following is a cycling parameter of mechanical ventilators?
  1. Volume
  2. Pressure
  3. Time
  4. Flow
     A. 1. and 2.
     B. 1. only
     C. 1., 2., and 3.
     D. All of the above

366. When a primary cycling parameter has been attained, which of the following is INCORRECT?
  A. An audio alarm will alarm
  B. A visual alarm will not alarm
  C. Inspiration will terminate
  D. None of the above

367. Which of the following are pressure-cycled ventilators?
  A. Bird Mark 7 and 8
  B. Bennett PR series
  C. Veriflo CV 2000
  D. Both A. and B.

368. Which of the following equipment have been identified as a causative agent of pneumonias from *Acinetobacter colcoaceticus*?
1. Wright respirometers
2. Wright peak flow meters
3. Bennett monitoring spirometers
4. Cascade humidifiers
   A. 1. only
   B. 4. only
   C. 1. and 3.
   D. 1. and 2.

369. Exhaled particles are sprayed from ventilators exhalation valves as far away as
A. 2 ft
B. 5 ft
C. 10 ft
D. 15 ft

370. A rule of thumb for estimating a patient's inspiratory peak flow rate is 4 to 6 times the measured
A. tidal volume
B. minute volume
C. vital capacity
D. negative inspiratory force

371. Which of the following has been named as relatively safe with regard to being a bacteria producer?
A. Spining disk nebulizer
B. Ultrasonic nebulizer
C. Cascade humidifier
D. Babbington nebulizer

372. The particulate water size produced by a nebulizer is
A. less than 5 μ
B. 5 to 8 μ
C. 8 to 12 μ
D. greater than 12 μ

Modes of Ventilation

DIRECTIONS (Questions 373–376): The group of questions below consists of a set of lettered items, followed by a list of numbered descriptions. Match each lettered item with the correct numbered description.

A. Control
B. Assist
C. Assist/Control
D. Intermittent Mandatory Ventilation (IMV)

373. The machine functions in the assist mode unless the patient's respiratory rate falls below a preset level, at which time the machine converts to the control mode.

374. The machine is responsible for initiation and delivery of each tidal volume.

375. The patient breathes spontaneously from an external high-flow system or from the ventilator via a demand valve, and at preset intervals the machine functions in the control mode.

376. The patient is totally responsible for initiation of the inspiratory phase, but the ventilator delivers the tidal volume.

DIRECTIONS (Questions 377–519): Each of the questions or incomplete statements below is followed by four suggested answers or completions. Select the **one** that is **best** in each case.

377. During pressure support mode ventilation, pressure develops rapidly in the ventilator system and remains at that level until spontaneous inspiratory flow rates decrease to what percent of peak inspiratory flow?
   A. 10%
   B. 15%
   C. 25%
   D. 30%

378. The patient is allowed to breath spontaneously from the ventilator via a demand valve, and at preset intervals the machine functions in the assist/control mode describes which of the following modes?
    A. CPAP
    B. SIMV
    C. IMV
    D. NEEP

379. Inspiratory airway maneuvers include
    A. sigh
    B. inflation hold
    C. flow taper
    D. all of the above

380. Which of the following are expiratory airway maneuvers?
    A. NEEP
    B. PEEP
    C. Expiratory retard
    D. All of the above

381. Which of the following ventilators have pneumatic powering mechanisms?
    1. Bird Mark 7
    2. Bennett PR-1
    3. Bear 1
    4. Puritan Bennett 7200
        A. 1. and 3.
        B. 1. and 2.
        C. 3. and 4.
        D. All of the above

382. Which of the following are double circuit ventilators?
    1. Emerson 3-PV IMV ventilator
    2. Bennett MA-1
    3. Bear 2
    4. Engstrom Erila
        A. 2. and 4.
        B. 2., 3., and 4.
        C. 1. and 3.
        D. All of the above

383. The Emerson 3-PV postoperative ventilator has which of the following gas flow and airway pressure patterns?
    A. Square wave flow with parabolic pressure pattern
    B. Sine wave and sigmoidal pressure pattern
    C. Sine wave with taper parabolic pressure pattern
    D. Accelerating flow with taper parabolic pressure pattern

384. Which of the following ventilators only offer PEEP as an expiratory airway maneuver?
    A. Bear 1
    B. MA-2
    C. MA-1
    D. A. and B.

385. Which of the following ventilators has a high/low oxygen percentage alarm incorporated from manufacture?
    A. Bennett MA-1
    B. Bear 1
    C. Servo 900C
    D. A. and C.

386. The limits on a Bear 1 ventilator include
    1. pressure
    2. flow
    3. time
    4. volume
        A. 1. and 2.
        B. 1. and 4.
        C. 3. and 4.
        D. 1., 2., and 3.

387. When the alarm silence is activated on a Bear 2 an audible alert/alarm will reactivate automatically in
    A. 30 sec
    B. 60 sec
    C. 90 sec
    D. 120 sec

388. On the Bear 2 when the sensitivity is set in the MORE position (5 o'clock), the patient must create a pressure drop greater than
   A. 0.5 cm H_2O at 2 L/min
   B. 1.0 cm H_2O at 2 L/min
   C. 1.0 cm H_2O at 5 L/min
   D. 0.5 cm H_2O at 5 L/min

389. On the Bear 2 when the oxygen % control is set above 21%, the audible/visual low O_2 pressure alert will be activated when inlet pressure drops below
   A. 27.5 + 2.5 psig
   B. 35 + 2.5 psig
   C. 40 + 2.5 psig
   D. 45 + 2.5 psig

390. The I:E ratio display is normally blank in which of the following modes on the Bear 2?
   A. SIMV
   B. CPAP
   C. Assist/control
   D. A. and B.

391. The maximum PEEP obtainable using the Bear 1 ventilator is
   A. 20 cm H_2O
   B. 30 cm H_2O
   C. 40 cm H_2O
   D. 50 cm H_2O

392. The Bear 1 and 2 ventilators will pressure limit correctly when the proximal airway pressure is indicating a
   A. higher value than set
   B. lower value than set
   C. equal value than is set
   D. none of the above

393. The tidal volume of the Bear 1 ventilator has a range of
   A. 0 to 2000 cc
   B. 100 to 2000 cc
   C. 50 to 2000 cc
   D. 100 to 2200 cc

394. The apnea alarm on the Bear 1 ventilator activates when the patient mechanical/spontaneous rate is less than:
    A. 5 breaths/min
    B. 4 breaths/min
    C. 3 breaths/min
    D. 2 breaths/min

395. Turning on the nebulizer on the Bear 1 ventilator will
    A. result in a higher tidal volume
    B. not affect the volume
    C. not change the FIO_2
    D. both B. and C.

396. The Bear 1 ventilator is PEEP-compensated in all modes of ventilation except
    A. control
    B. assist/control
    C. SIMV
    D. none of the above

397. During the application of PEEP using the Bear 1, a patient circuit disconnect will induce a continuous flow from the demand valve of up to
    A. 90 L/min
    B. 100 L/min
    C. 110 L/min
    D. 120 L/min

398. When using the nebulizer on the MA-1, the tidal volume and oxygen will
    A. both increase
    B. not change
    C. volume increases, oxygen remains the same
    D. oxygen increases, volume remains the same

399. The approximate maximum PEEP level obtainable by the MA-1 ventilator is
    A. 15 cm H_2O
    B. 25 cm H_2O
    C. 30 cm H_2O
    D. 35 cm H_2O

400. The tidal volume range of the MA-1 ventilator is
    A. 100 to 2200 cc
    B. 0 to 2000 cc
    C. 0 to 2200 cc
    D. 100 to 2000 cc

401. The controlled rate range of the MA-1 ventilator is
    A. 6 to 60 cycles/min
    B. 0 to 60 cycles/min
    C. 6 to 80 cycles/min
    D. 0 to 100 cycles/min

402. When using PEEP/CPAP, which of the following is not correct?
    A. Maintains lung volumes at more normal levels
    B. Reduces intrapulmonary shunting and hypoxemia
    C. Compliance improves
    D. Airway resistance increases

403. Long-term mechanical ventilation generally requires a ventilator capable of
    A. high pressure and flow characteristics
    B. high pressure and low flow characteristics
    C. low pressure and high flow characteristics
    D. low pressure and flow characteristics

404. Which of the following is not a required control parameter when placing the Bear 5 in the AMV mode?
    A. Tidal volume
    B. Peak flow
    C. Rate
    D. Minimum MV

405. The normal rate parameter range of the Bear 5 is:
    A. 0 to 150 breaths/min
    B. 5 to 120 breaths/min
    C. 1 to 120 breaths/min
    D. 0 to 100 breaths/min

406. The maximum sigh volume which can be set on the Bear 5 is
- **A.** 2000 cc
- **B.** 2500 cc
- **C.** 3000 cc
- **D.** 3500 cc

407. The peak flow parameter range of the Bear 5 is
- **A.** 10 to 100 L/min
- **B.** 10 to 120 L/min
- **C.** 5 to 120 L/min
- **D.** 5 to 150 L/min

408. Pressure support is not available in which of the following modes on the Bear 5?
- **A.** AMV
- **B.** SIMV
- **C.** IMV
- **D.** Time cycle

409. Which of the following is the only mechanical control adjustment on the Bennett 7200?
- **A.** Respiratory rate
- **B.** High/low pressure alarm
- **C.** Low PEEP/CPAP alarm
- **D.** PEEP/CPAP setting

410. The Bennett 7200 offers which of the following flow wave forms?
- **A.** Square
- **B.** Tapered
- **C.** Sine
- **D.** All of the above

411. Given the following information, the calculated ventilator circuit compliance is
Given: Volume of gas leaving manifold: 240 mL
     End-expiratory pressure: 0 cm H_2O
     Occluded peak pressure: 60 cm H_2O
  A. 6 mL/cm H_2O
  B. 5 mL/cm H_2O
  C. 4 mL/cm H_2O
  D. 3 mL/cm H_2O

412. The primary use of pressure-cycled ventilators today is
  A. preterm infant
  B. recovery room ventilation
  C. intermittent positive pressure breathing treatments (IPPB)
  D. all of the above

413. The time-cycled, pressure-preset type ventilators are used most frequently for
  A. preterm infant
  B. muscular deficiency patients
  C. recovery room ventilation
  D. IPPB

414. Which of the following ventilators have a combined electric/pneumatic powering mechanism?
  A. Bourns BP200
  B. Sechrist IV-100B
  C. Healthdyne 105
  D. All of the above

415. The Bourns BP300 has which of the following modes of ventilation?
  A. IMV
  B. CPAP
  C. Assist
  D. Both A. and B.

416. The Bourns BP200 has which of the following gas flow and pressure patterns?
   A. Square wave flow and rectilinear pressure pattern
   B. Accelerating flow and nonlinear pressure pattern
   C. Decelerating flow and parabolic pressure pattern
   D. Decelerating flow and rectilinear pressure pattern

417. The flow range of the Sechrist IV-100B infant ventilator is
   A. 0 to 32 L/min flush to 40 L/min
   B. 0 to 40 L/min flush to 50 L/min
   C. 0 to 50 L/min
   D. 0 to 55 L/min

418. The inspiratory pressure range of the Sechrist IV-100B infant ventilator is
   A. 0 to 50 cm H_2O
   B. 5 to 60 cm H_2O
   C. 7 to 70 cm H_2O
   D. 7 to 80 cm H_2O

419. The alarm delay time of the Sechrist IV-100B infant ventilator is
   A. 3 to 20 sec $\pm$ 10%
   B. 5 to 30 sec $\pm$ 10%
   C. 3 to 50 sec $\pm$ 10%
   D. 3 to 60 sec $\pm$ 10%

420. The safety pressure pop-off is adjusted by
   A. occluding the patient connection and the exhalation tube simultaneously
   B. setting flow rate at 5 L/min
   C. reading the pressure on the manometer
   D. all of the above

421. The normal exhalation valve supplied with the Sechrist IV-100B infant ventilator is designed to work best in a flow range of approximately
   A. 3 to 12 L/min
   B. 3 to 30 L/min
   C. 5 to 40 L/min
   D. 5 to 50 L/min

422. The pediatric exhalation valve is designed to be used for flows up to approximately
A. 40 L/min
B. 50 L/min
C. 60 L/min
D. 70 L/min

423. The set point indicator for the ventilator monitor alarm on the Sechrist IV-100B should be set
A. 1 to 2 cm H_2O above the maximum pressure
B. 3 to 4 cm H_2O below the maximum pressure
C. 1 to 2 cm H_2O below the maximum pressure
D. 3 to 4 cm H_2O above the maximum pressure

424. The wave form of the Healthdyne 100 ventilator is dependent on which of the following?
A. Flow
B. Inspiratory time
C. Pressure limit
D. All of the above

425. The respiratory rate is adjusted on the Healthdyne 100 ventilator from
A. 0 to 100
B. 0 to 80
C. 0 to 60
D. 0 to 50

426. The minimum expiratory time of the Healthdyne 100 ventilator is
A. 0.3 sec
B. 0.5 sec
C. 0.7 sec
D. 1.0 sec

427. The PEEP/CPAP range of the Healthdyne 100 ventilator is
A. 0 to 20 cm H_2O
B. 0 to 25 cm H_2O
C. 0 to 30 cm H_2O
D. 0 to 35 cm H_2O

428. The pressure limit is adjustable on the Healthdyne 100 ventilator from
    A. 1 to 100 cm H_2O
    B. 1 to 70 cm H_2O
    C. 1 to 50 cm H_2O
    D. 5 to 50 cm H_2O

429. The Bio-Med Devices MVP-10 ventilator is intended primarily for tidal volumes in the range up to
    A. 300 mL
    B. 400 mL
    C. 500 mL
    D. 1000 mL

430. The respiratory rate of the MVP-10 ventilator is variable from
    A. 0 to 80
    B. 0 to 100
    C. 0 to 120
    D. 0 to 150

431. The safety relief valve on the MVP-10 opens at
    A. −2 cm H_2O
    B. −4 cm H_2O
    C. −8 cm H_2O
    D. −10 cm H_2O

432. When using the MVP-10 for transports in nonpressurized aircraft the actual inspiratory and expiratory times will
    A. increase by 1½% for every 1000
    B. Increase by 2½% for every 1000
    C. not be affected
    D. the unit cannot be used as a transport ventilator

433. Which of the following is not true about High-Frequency Ventilation (HFV)?
    A. Tidal volumes may be less than anatomical deadspace
    B. Peak inflation pressure is much higher than conventional mechanical ventilation
    C. mean airway pressure may be lower
    D. frequency may exceed 1000 breaths/min

434. Which of the following are advantages of HFV?
   A. Lower incidence of pulmonary baratrauma
   B. Less cardiovascular depression
   C. Reduced mechanical deadspace
   D. Both A. and B.

435. Proposed explanations for the mechanisms of gas transport with HFV include
   A. Brownian motion
   B. convection
   C. augmented transport
   D. all of the above

436. High-Frequency Positive-Pressure Ventilation (HFPPV) uses frequencies and tidal volumes of
   A. frequency 60 to 90; volumes 200 to 300 mL
   B. frequency 100 to 150; volumes 100 to 200 mL
   C. frequency 150 to 500; volumes 100 to 200 mL
   D. frequency 500 to 1000; volumes 200 to 300 mL

437. High-Frequency Jet Ventilation (HFJV) uses breathing rates per minute of
   A. 100 to 150
   B. 100 to 500
   C. 100 to 900
   D. 500 to 1000

438. The optimal inspiratory time setting for gas exchange with HFPPV appears to be
   A. 22% of the respiratory cycle
   B. 35% of the respiratory cycle
   C. 50% of the respiratory cycle
   D. 60% of the respiratory cycle

439. Reported complications of HFJV include
1. inadequate humidification
2. damage to tracheal mucosa
3. bronchopleural fistula
4. pneumothorax
   A. 1. only
   B. 1. and 3.
   C. 1. and 2.
   D. all of the above

440. When using infusion as the means for humidification for HFJV, the normal rate is
   A. 10 to 20 mL/hr
   B. 20 to 30 mL/hr
   C. 30 to 40 mL/hr
   D. 40 to 50 mL/hr

441. High-Frequency Oscillation (HFO) has been successfully used at frequencies ranging from
   A. 500 to 1000 breaths/min
   B. 1000 to 1500 breaths/min
   C. 1500 to 2000 breaths/min
   D. 900 to 3000 breaths/min

442. The tidal volumes of HFO have been estimated to range from
   A. 5 to 50 mL
   B. 5 to 80 mL
   C. 50 to 100 mL
   D. 25 to 100 mL

443. The using HFJV which of the following will not decrease arterial Pco_2?
   A. increasing driving pressure
   B. increasing % TI at a constant RR
   C. increasing RR at a constant % TI
   D. increasing jet diameter

444. Inadvertent PEEP with High-Frequency Ventilation is a result of
  A. compliance and resistance of patient and tubing
  B. frequency and percent inspiratory time dependent
  C. increased expiratory time with increased gas inflows
  D. driving pressure set too high

445. Noninvasive ventilatory support devices include all of the following, except
  A. Pulmo-wrap
  B. rocking bed
  C. LP-6
  D. chest cuirass

446. Which of the following portable ventilators, which are primarily used in the home, have a fixed I:E ratio?
  A. Life Products LP-3
  B. Life Products LP-4
  C. Thompson M25B
  D. Life Products LP-5

447. For the patient discharged to home on a ventilator, which of the following would NOT be required?
  A. Manual resuscitator
  B. Suction machine
  C. Heart monitor
  D. Air compressor

448. Which of the following should be monitored on ventilators?
  1. Electronic source
  2. Pneumatic sources
  3. Inspiratory/expiratory gas composition
  4. Inspired gas temperature
  5. Respiratory rate
      A. 2., 4., and 5.
      B. 1., 2., and 3.
      C. 2., 3., 4., and 5.
      D. All of the above

449. An electrical power failure monitor should provide a sufficient audible tone that
   A. can be heard from a distance of 20 yd
   B. lasts for at least 5 min
   C. has a different tone than any other alarm
   D. is accompanied by a visible alarm

450. Activation of the oxygen source failure alarm on a mechanical ventilator indicates
   A. increase in FIO_2 that is set
   B. decrease in FIO_2 that is set
   C. insufficient oxygen pressure
   D. all of the above

451. A polarographic cell works on the same principle as
   A. Clark electrode
   B. Severinghaus electrode
   C. thermal conductivity
   D. ionization

452. When an oxygen monitor is engaged continuously, recalibration should be completed how frequently?
   A. At least every 8 hr
   B. At least every 12 hr
   C. At least every 16 hr
   D. Once a day

453. If a polarographic oxygen monitor is calibrated at ambient pressure and is placed on a ventilator, the actual display is
   A. lower than the FIO_2
   B. not affected by pressure
   C. higher than the FIO_2
   D. correct because the monitor corrects for increased pressure

454. Theoretically the oxygen monitor reading will be incorrect by
   A. 1% per 10 cm H_2O above atmospheric pressure
   B. 2% per 10 cm H_2O above atmospheric pressure
   C. 3% per 10 cm H_2O above atmospheric pressure
   D. 4% per 10 cm H_2O above atmospheric pressure

455. When an oxygen monitor is placed into a environment of 100% relative humidity at 37°C, the display will
   A. not be affected
   B. be higher
   C. be lower
   D. vary

456. The theoretical decrease in displayed oxygen concentration due to humidity is
   A. 1%
   B. 2%
   C. 3%
   4. 4%

457. Capnometers measure CO_2 levels by
   A. Severinghaus principle
   B. infrared analyzer
   C. Clark electrode
   D. ionization

458. A mass spectrometer distinguishes different gas samples according to
   A. atomic particle charge
   B. radiation absorption
   C. ionic charge
   D. molecular valance

459. Phase 1 of the carbon dioxide wave form (capnogram) represents
   A. mixture of deadspace and "alveolar" gas
   B. arterial P_{CO_2}
   C. "alveolar" carbon dioxide concentration
   D. gas that remained in the deadspace at the end of the preceding inspiration

460. Phase 2 of the capnogram represents
   A. mixture of deadspace and "alveolar" gas
   B. arterial P_{CO_2}
   C. "alveolar" carbon dioxide concentration
   D. gas that remained in the deadspace at the end of the preceding inspiration

461. Phase 3 of the capnogram represents
   A. mixture of deadspace and "alveolar" gas
   B. arterial P_{CO_2}
   C. "alveolar" carbon dioxide concentration
   D. gas that remained in the deadspace at the end of the preceding inspiration

462. In the normal individual the peak expired Pet_{CO_2} is
   A. equal to the arterial P_{CO_2}.
   B. 1 to 10 mmHg greater than the arterial P_{CO_2}.
   C. 1 to 7 mmHg less than the arterial P_{CO_2}.
   D. 5 to 15 mmHg less than the arterial P_{CO_2}.

463. Mainstream transducers and sample ports of aspirating capnometers must be placed
   A. in expiratory line of the patient circuit
   B. between the patient airway and the breathing circuit
   C. after the exhalation port
   D. before any humidification device

464. The plateau of the capnogram represents
   A. exhalation phase
   B. inhalation phase
   C. end-exhalation and respiratory pause
   D. alveolar plateau

465. When using transcutaneous oxygen monitoring (Ptc_{O_2}), the electrode must be allowed to stabilize for how long before clinical use?
   A. 10 min
   B. 20 min
   C. 30 min
   D. 40 min

466. The Ptc_{O_2}
   A. is equal to arterial PO_2
   B. is higher than arterial PO_2
   C. is lower than arterial PO_2
   D. correlates to arterial PO_2

467. The movement of the Ptco$_2$ electrode is required
   A. to allow the tissue to be reoxygenated
   B. to prevent mild burns
   C. to improve arterial correlation
   D. all of the above

468. Accuracy of Ptco$_2$ can be impaired by which of the following?
   1. Hypotension
   2. Obesity
   3. Acidosis
   4. Certain anesthetics
      A. 1. and 2.
      B. 1. and 3.
      C. 2. and 3.
      D. All of the above

469. When using pulse oximetry, the measurement may be impaired in heavy smokers by
   A. carboxyhemoglobin
   B. hyperoxin
   C. desaturation
   D. hypoxia

470. The Ohio Pediatric Aerosol Tent is designed
   A. to provide a water-saturated atmosphere that will have sufficient cooling to lower the canopy temperature
   B. to provide an oxygen-enriched environment
   C. specifically for the treatment of asthma
   D. all of the above

471. The Ohio Pediatric Aerosol Tent, when placed in the cool mode, will lower the temperature by which of the following ranges of below ambient temperature?
   A. 4°F to 5°F
   B. 6°F to 15°F
   C. 8°F to 20°F
   D. 10°F to 25°F

472. The Ohio High-Output Pneumatic Nebulizer is capable of nebulizing up to
     A. 2 cc/min
     B. 4 cc/min
     C. 6 cc/min
     D. 8 cc/min

473. To avoid buildup of excess carbon dioxide in the tent canopy, a minimum liter flow of _____ is required
     A. 5 L/min
     B. 10 L/min
     C. 15 L/min
     D. 20 L/min

474. The Laerdal Bag Mask Resuscitator for children and infants has a pressure-limiting safety valve which is preset at
     A. 40 cm H_2O
     B. 45 cm H_2O
     C. 50 cm H_2O
     D. 55 cm H_2O

475. The Puritan PMR2 Resuscitator has a preset safety valve on all units set at
     A. 40 cm H_2O
     B. 45 cm H_2O
     C. 50 cm H_2O
     D. 55 cm H_2O

476. The maximum FIO_2 provided by the Laerdal Resuscitator is
     A. 0.80
     B. 0.90
     C. 0.95
     D. 1.00

477. The volume of the Laerdal Adult Resuscitator Bag is
     A. 2200 cc
     B. 2000 cc
     C. 1600 cc
     D. 1000 cc

478. The volume of the Laerdal Child Resuscitator Bag is
   A. 240 mL
   B. 500 mL
   C. 750 mL
   D. 1200 mL

479. The volume of the Laerdal Infant Resuscitator Bag is
   A. 100 mL
   B. 150 mL
   C. 240 mL
   D. 400 mL

480. The volume of the reservoir bag for the adult and child Laerdal Resuscitator is
   A. 2600 mL
   B. 2000 mL
   C. 1600 mL
   D. 1000 mL

481. The volume of the reservoir bag for the infant Laerdal Resuscitator is
   A. 240 mL
   B. 400 mL
   C. 600 mL
   D. 800 mL

482. Endotracheal tubes for neonates to adults range in length from
   A. 6 cm to 18 cm
   B. 9 cm to 28 cm
   C. 12 cm to 38 cm
   D. 15 cm to 48 cm

483. The internal diameter of endotracheal tubes for neonates to adults range from
   A. 2.5 mm to 11 mm
   B. 5 mm to 16 mm
   C. 7.5 mm to 21 mm
   D. 10 mm to 26 mm

484. The most commonly used plastic for artificial airways is
  A. silicone
  B. polyethylene
  C. teflon
  D. polyvinyl chloride

485. All tubes used for airway management should have which of the following markings?
  1. Z-79 and/or IT
  2. Internal diameter
  3. Type of cuff
  4. Tubing length
  5. External diameter
    A. 1., 2., and 4.
    B. 1. only
    C. 1., 2., 4., and 5.
    D. All of the above

486. The IT on endotracheal tubes stands for
  A. intubation tube
  B. implantation tube
  C. implantation testing
  D. inhalation therapy

487. The preferred cuff on a tracheal device has which of the following characteristics?
  A. high-volume, high-pressure
  B. high-volume, low-pressure
  C. low-volume, low-pressure
  D. low-volume, high-pressure

488. The curved blade used with the laryngoscope is also called
  A. Miller
  B. MacGyver
  C. McGill
  D. MacIntosh

489. The straight blade used with the laryngoscope is also called
  A. Miller
  B. MacGyver
  C. McGill
  D. MacIntosh

490. The long-nosed forceps is used during intubation to
    A. hold tongue away from airway
    B. lift epiglottis
    C. guide nasotracheal tube into trachea
    D. all of the above

491. When using a stylet during intubation, the distal end of the rod should be
    A. at the end of the tube
    B. ½ in. from the end of the tube
    B. 2 in. from the end of the tube
    D. one-half the length of the tube

492. Tracheal capillary blood pressure is about
    A. 15 mmHg
    B. 25 mmHg
    C. 35 mmHg
    D. 45 mmHg

493. Cuff inflation pressures should be checked
    A. each time the cuff is inflated
    B. every 4 hr
    C. every 8 hr
    D. A. and C.

494. Tracheostomy tubes vary in length from
    A. 2 to 4 in.
    B. 2 to 6 in.
    C. 3 to 8 in.
    D. 4 to 8 in.

495. The internal diameter of a tracheostomy tube ranges from
    A. 2 to 12 mm
    B. 3 to 14 mm
    C. 4 to 16 mm
    D. 6 to 15 mm

496. Permanent tracheostomy tubes are made of
    A. stainless steel
    B. aluminum
    C. silver
    D. all of the above

497. Tracheostomy buttons are used for
  A. maintaining stoma patency
  B. allowing gradual stoma closure
  C. weaning
  D. all of the above

498. Without the tracheostomy button in place, the stoma would close within
  A. 24 to 36 hr
  B. 32 to 48 hr
  C. 48 to 72 hr
  D. 56 to 84 hr

499. The inner cannula of a double cannula tracheostomy tube should be cleaned at least every
  A. 4 hr
  B. 8 hr
  C. 12 hr
  D. 24 hr

500. The inner cannula is cleaned using
  A. 0.25% acetic acid solution
  B. mild soap
  C. 2% hydrogen peroxide
  D. Cidex

501. When performing intubation the laryngoscope is held in
  A. the left hand
  B. the right hand
  C. either hand
  D. it varies with the type of blade

502. The safe therapeutic range for tracheal aspiration in the pediatric patient is
  A. 40 to 60 mmHg
  B. 60 to 80 mmHg
  C. 80 to 120 mmHg
  D. 120 to 150 mmHg

503. The safe therapeutic range for tracheal aspiration in the neonatal patient is
   A. 40 to 60 mmHg
   B. 60 to 80 mmHg
   C. 80 to 120 mmHg
   D. 120 to 150 mmHg

504. Connection tubing and reservoir jars from the vacuum equipment to the suction catheter should be changed at least every
   A. 72 hr
   B. 48 hr
   C. 24 hr
   D. 8 hr

505. For successful completion of the suctioning procedure, the patient should be placed in
   A. semi-Fowler's position
   B. prone
   C. Fowler's
   D. Trendelenburg

506. Prior to suctioning, a patient receiving oxygen should be administered 100% oxygen for at least
   A. 5 breaths
   B. 30 sec
   C. 1 min
   D. 5 min

507. Which of the following is INCORRECT about suctioning procedures?
   A. The catheter should be inserted into the airway as far as it will advance
   B. Suction should be applied continuously while withdrawing the catheter
   C. The catheter should be rotated 360 deg. between the fingers as it is withdrawn.
   D. The total procedure from insertion to complete withdrawal should take no more than 20 sec.

508. Oxygen concentrations in tents range from
   A. 30% to 50%
   B. 40% to 60%
   C. 50% to 70%
   D. 60% to 80%

509. Oxygen percentage of an oxygen hood may be as high as
   A. 60%
   B. 75%
   C. 90%
   D. 100%

510. The Wheatstone Bridge principle of oxygen analyzing is the same as
   A. paramagnetic principle
   B. thermal conductivity
   C. galvanic cell
   D. polarographic electrode

511. The particle size generated by the SPAG-2 is
   A. 95% less than 5 μ diameter
   B. 80% less than 7 μ diameter
   C. 90% less than 2 μ diameter
   D. 85% less than 6 μ diameter

512. When administering virazole, the drug must be mixed with
   A. a bronchodilator
   B. a mucolytic agent
   C. 300 mL sterile water for injection or inhalation
   D. 300 mL normal saline solution

513. The SPAG-2 requires an operating pressure of
   A. 26 psig
   B. 35 psig
   C. 45 psig
   D. 50 psig

514. The flow rate range of the SPAG-2 is
   A. 5 to 8 L/min
   B. 8 to 12 L/min
   C. 12.5 to 15 L/min
   D. 15.5 to 20.5 L/min

515. Reconstituted solutions of virazole may be stored under sterile conditions, at room temperature for
    A. 12 hr
    B. 24 hr
    C. 48 hr
    D. 72 hr

516. Virazole solutions which have been placed in the SPAG-2 units should be discarded at least every
    A. 12 hr
    B. 24 hr
    C. 48 hr
    D. 72 hr

517. The administration of virazole is carried out for
    A. 12 to 18 hr/day for a minimum of 3 days
    B. 16 to 24 hr/day for a minimum of 5 days
    C. 10 to 15 hr/day for a minimum of 7 days
    D. 8 to 12 hr/day for a minimum of 3 days

518. The recommended delivery mechanism for virazole is
    A. face mask
    B. infant oxygen hood
    C. oxygen/humidity tent
    D. ventilator

519. Virazole should not be administered for more than
    A. 5 days
    B. 7 days
    C. 10 days
    D. 14 days

Explanatory Answers

289. B. The capacity an oxygen E-cylinder will hold is 22 ft². 12.7 ft² of oxygen will occupy a D-cylinder while 28 ft² and 32 ft² will overfill or underfill the remaining cylinder sizes. (**Ref.** 22, p. 360)

290. C. An H or K size oxygen cylinder will hold 244 ft² of gas, while a G-cylinder will hold 187 ft² of oxygen. (**Ref.** 22, p. 360)

291. C. The maximum filling pressure for an oxygen cylinder is 2200 psi, regardless of the cylinder size. (**Ref.** 22, p. 360)

292. B. 2.41 is the multiplication factor utilized with G-cylinders. 3.14 is for H-cylinders. To determine this number an equation can be expressed as

$$\text{Factor} = \frac{(\text{cubic volume}) \ (28.3 \ \text{L/ft}^2)}{2200 \ \text{psi}}$$

(**Ref.** 22, p. 360)

293. A. Cylinder duration can be expressed as

$$\text{Time} = \frac{(\text{Gauge pressure}) \ (\text{Multiplication factor})}{\text{liter flow} \times 60}$$

So that

$$\frac{(1500) \times (.28 \ \text{for E-cycle})}{4 \ \text{L/min} \times 60 \ \text{min}} = \frac{420}{240} = 1.75 \ \text{hr}$$

(**Ref.** 22, p. 360)

294. A. The factor for an H-cylinder is 3.14. If the present pressure is 1400 psi and the patient changes it at 200 psi then the working pressure is 1200; therefore,

$$\frac{1200 \ \text{psi} \times 3.14}{6 \ \text{L/min} \times 60 \ \text{min}} = \frac{3768}{360} = 10.5 \ \text{hr}$$

(**Ref.** 22, p. 360)

295. C. High-pressure gas regulators reduce cylinder pressures to a usable working pressure of 50 psi. (**Ref.** 22, p. 361)

296. C. A single-stage regulator incorporates a preset safety pop-off that operates at a pressure of 200 psi. (**Ref.** 22, p. 362)

297. A. Bourdon gauges are pressure-sensitive devices that utilize expandable copper coils to indicate pressure and flow. Any resistance added distal to the gauge will create back pressure, thereby causing higher than actual readings for flow. Thorpe tubes use needle valves and floats as opposed to a coil. (**Ref.** 22, p. 364)

298. D. With a noncompensated Thorpe tube, the flow control is located proximal to the inlet pressure so that the float is calibrated to atmospheric pressure. When back pressure is applied the float will read lower than the actual gas flow output of the device. Bourdon gauges read higher outputs in the face of back pressure, while compensated Thorpe tubes will retain accuracy despite resistance to flow. (**Ref.** 22, p. 365)

299. C. The flow control on a compensated Thorpe tube is located between the float and output. In this situation, since the float is always exposed to and calibrated a 50 psi gas source, back pressure will have no effect on the flow indicator since back pressure cannot exceed 50 psi. (**Ref.** 28, p. 136)

300. B. To maintain accuracy, flowmeters are calibrated to a working pressure of 45.55 psig. They must not be used when pressures exceed the 50 ± 5 psig variance. (**Ref.** 28, p. 134)

301. D. Accuracy of flowmeters is determined by these factors: the device must be in an upright position, it must be used with the appropriate inlet pressure (50 ± 5 psig) and the valve seat must be intact or leakage will occur into the room. (**Ref.** 28, p. 135)

302. B. Bourdon flowmeters are most accurate in a flow range of 3 to 7 L/min. In lower flows there is a 10% error factor. Accuracy at all flows is compromised by back pressure. (**Ref.** 28, p. 136)

303. A. Generally oxygen delivery devices are subdivided into low-flow and high-flow systems. Demand and closed systems can actually be subdivisions of low- and high-flow delivery devices. (**Ref.** 22, p. 375)

304. C. Low-flow systems result in an unpredictable and extremely variable FIO_2. Factors affecting delivery include gas flow, patient's minute volume, and the type of equipment used. (**Ref.** 22, p. 377)

305. B. Since low-flow devices typically do not meet patients' flow demands, any increase in minute volume will result in further entrainment of room air with a decrease in FIO_2. (**Ref.** 22, p. 378)

306. B. The rule of thumb for FIO_2 delivered by nasal cannulas can be expressed as follows. For each liter of flow, add 4% oxygen to 20%. Therefore, a 4 L flow would result in 20% + 16% = 36% FIO_2. It must be stressed that this is dependent on the patient's inspiratory demands. (**Ref.** 22, p. 379)

307. B. Simple face masks should be operated at flows of 5 to 8 L/min. This flow is needed to ensure the prevention of CO_2 accumulation. (**Ref.** 22, p. 379)

308. B. A flow rate of 5 to 8 L/min will result in a delivered FIO_2 of 40% to 60% which is dependent on the patient's breathing pattern. (**Ref.** 22, p. 379)

309. B. A partial rebreather should be run at a liter flow of 7 to 10 L/min. This should be titrated to ensure the bag deflates approximately one-third during inspiration. CO_2 buildup may occur should the bag collapse greater than one-third. (**Ref.** 22, p. 379)

310. C. The FIO_2 delivered by a partial rebreather with the proper flow setting is between 70% and 80%, depending on the patient's respiratory pattern. (**Ref.** 22, p. 379)

311. C. Nonrebreathing generally can be operated at flows of 8 to 10 L/min. However, proper use is to ensure the reservoir bag never completely collapses during inspiration. (**Ref.** 28, p. 265)

312. C. Use of flows in excess of 6 L/min via a nasal cannula often poses discomfort to a patient and results in mucosal irritation. Oxygen toxicity and FIO_2 above 50% are generally not associated with low-flow devices. (**Ref.** 28, p. 257)

313. C. Recently, studies have demonstrated that at flows of 4 L/min or less, artificial humidification is not indicated. (**Ref.** 28, p. 257)

314. C. In situations where patients breathe extremely shallow, FIO_2 can even approach 90% FIO_2. Other hazards include a decrease in ventilation in patients with severe COPD and, as always, the potential for fire whenever oxygen is used. Contrary to popular belief, nasal cannulas are effective in patients who breathe through their mouths. (**Ref.** 28, p. 258)

315. D. Care must be taken not to assume the accuracy of FIO_2 delivered by some venturi masks. Studies indicate that venturi devices may be in error by as much as 8%. (**Ref.** 28, p. 260)

316–319. Although entrainment ratios should be memorized, an equation that can be used to determine approximate entrainment ratios can be expressed as

$$\frac{100 - FIO_2}{FIO_2 - 20} = \text{Liters of air} : \text{Liters of O}_2$$

(**Ref.** 28, p. 262)

316. C. $\dfrac{100 - 24\%}{24 - 20} = \dfrac{76}{4} = 19:1 \text{ or } @ \ 20:1$

317. B. $\dfrac{100 - 28\%}{28 - 20} = \dfrac{72}{8} = 9:1 \text{ or } @ \ 10:1$

318. D. $\dfrac{100 - 35\%}{35 - 20} = \dfrac{65}{15} = 4.3:1 \text{ or } @ \ 5:1$

319. A. $\dfrac{100 - 40\%}{40 - 20} = \dfrac{60}{10} = 3:1$

320. D. With the use of nasal oxygen catheters, care should be taken to alternate nares every 12 to 24 hr to minimize mucosal irritation. (**Ref.** 42, p. 141)

321. B. With little increase in oxygen capacitance, simple face masks offer little improvement over the use of nasal cannulas or nasal catheters. (**Ref.** 42, p. 140)

322. C. Most commercially available bubble humidifiers will increase the relative humidity up to 80% to 90% at ambient temperatures by splitting the gas into tiny bubbles, thereby increasing the surface area of the gas that is exposed to liquid. (**Ref.** 42, p. 141)

323. A. A humidity deficit will occur at inspired water contents less than 43.8 mg/L. The amount of mucosal evaporation is directly related to the deficit which will result in increased mucus viscosity. (**Ref.** 42, p. 141)

324. D. With the deficit in water content, humidity deficit will result in a chain reaction beginning with mucosal dehydration, increased viscosity of the mucus, then decreased mucociliary clearance. (**Ref.** 42, p. 141)

325. D. Although humidifiers provide 80% to 90% of relative humidity at ambient temperature, once the gas is warmed to body temperature the relative humidity decreases to 30% to 40%. (**Ref.** 28, p. 285)

326. A. Insertion of a nasal catheter should be estimated by the distance measured from the patient's nose to the tragus of the ear. After insertion the tip of the catheter may be viewed just behind the uvula. (**Ref.** 28, p. 260)

327. C. Depending on the frequency generated, ultrasonic nebulizers produce particles in the size range of 1 to 10 μ. (**Ref.** 28, p. 305)

328. A. Ultrasonic nebulizers on the average will produce particles of 3 μ at a range of 1 to 10 μ. (**Ref.** 28, p. 305)

329. C. Because of inherent restrictions in the outflow of jet nebulizers, total oxygen flow rates cannot exceed 14 to 16 L/min at 50 psi. This situation becomes critical as the patient's inspired flow rates exceed the flow delivered by the jet nebulizer. This results in increased air entrainment and decreased delivered FIO_2. (**Ref.** 42, p. 142)

330. C. Ultrasonic nebulizers produce aerosol particles by the use of sound waves produced by a piezoelectric crystal vibrating at a frequency of 1.35 mHz. (**Ref.** 28, p. 305)

331. A. Mechanical nebulizers produce outputs of 1 to 1.5 mL/min, with 55% of the particles falling within the therapeutic range of 1 to 5 μ. (**Ref.** 22, p. 394)

332. B. Babington nebulizers produce an output of approximately 6 mL/min. 50% of their output falls within therapeutic range (1 to 5 μ). (**Ref.** 22, p. 395)

333. C. Ultrasonic nebulizers far exceed the therapeutic outputs of most other aerosol generators by producing particles of 1 to 5 μ 97% of the time. The Bird, Puritan Bennett, and Babington nebulizers only reach about 50% to 55% efficiency. (**Ref.** 22, p. 395)

334. C. With the proliferation of disposable equipment, Babington nebulizers have become "dinosaurs" in the history of respiratory equipment. They can be easily identified by their small hollow glass spheres. (**Ref.** 20, p. 294)

335. D. The Monaghan 225, Sechrist IV-100B, and Ohio 550 ventilators all incorporate the use of fluidic logic in their operation. (**Ref.** 22, p. 432)

336. A. The Coanda effect principally describes the use of fluidics in ventilation. It is described as the effect that a free-flowing gas creates a subatmospheric pressure at this periphery. This negative pressure causes a stream of gas to adhere to a wall. (**Ref.** 22, p. 423)

337. D. Streams of gas influenced by principles of fluidics can be changed directionally by either back pressure, subatmospheric pressure, or amplification. (**Ref.** 22, p. 423)

338. B. Endotracheal suctioning should only be performed when indicated so as to minimize trauma to the respiratory tract mucosa. It should never be performed routinely or prophylactically, as it predisposes patients to significant hypoxemia. (**Ref.** 42, p. 143)

339. D. Respiratory tract mucosa, when exposed to the hazards of tracheal suctioning may elicit trauma in the form of mucosal erosion hemorrhage and depression of the mucociliary transport mechanisms. There is also a resultant predisposition for bacterial colonization. More acute effects may include hypoxemia and bradycardia. (**Ref.** 42, p. 143)

340. A. When tracheal suction is performed, negative pressure should not be applied for greater than 15 sec. A common rule of thumb is to hold your breath during the procedure so as to mimic the effect of breathlessness you inflict on the patient. (**Ref.** 42, p. 143)

341. C. When performing direct tracheal suctioning, hyperoxygenation should be applied prior to and following the procedure. This practice will minimize the hypoxia caused by the procedure to patients who breathe secondary to hypoxic drive.

342. B. Suction catheters should not exceed one-half the diameter of the airway to be suctioned. This prevents total occlusion of the airway and affords the patient the ability to exchange gas. Although transparency in catheters may be desired, it is not necessary. The length of catheters should vary to accommodate differences in airways as well as the sizes of patients. (**Ref.** 42, p. 143)

343. D. IPPB may be used in patients in which spontaneous ventilation is inadequate to deliver medication to the site of action within the lungs. It also improves coughing and expectoration by forcing air below areas occupied by mucus. It also provides for the elimination of CO_2, thereby decreasing the $PaCO_2$ and relieving patients of pulmonary distress. (**Ref.** 43, p. 148)

344. C. Since IPPB therapy is prescribed to facilitate deep breaths, tidal volumes should be measured to assess the adequacy of therapy. To be of benefit, volumes should exceed the maximum inspired volume by at least 25%. (**Ref.** 43, p. 148)

345. C. If a patient's postoperative vital capacity is within 10% to 20% of his/her preoperative vital capacity, IPPB therapy may not be indicated. (**Ref.** 43, p. 148)

346. D. The success of sustained maximal inspiration therapy lies in factors that include knowledge of the preoperative base line, volume, and the duration of end-inspiratory hold. Recent studies have demonstrated that incentive breathing is at least as effective as IPPB therapy. (**Ref.** 43, p. 149)

347. D. In order to prevent aspiration of secretions, the following procedures must be carried out if it is necessary to deflate the cuff of an artificial airway:
1. suction the trachea
2. suction the area above the cuff as well as possible through the pharynx
3. follow with trachea suctioning after cuff deflation. (**Ref.** 5, p. 266)

348. C. Postural drainage often results in the patient being able to produce a sputum specimen suitable for culture. Rinsing catheters with normal saline and obtaining specimens after trach care may invalidate the sample obtained. (**Ref.** 5, p. 262)

349. D. Suction catheters should never be advanced with suction applied, as this will result in tracheal damage.. When suctioning is performed, the catheter should not be left in the airway for longer than 15 sec. Finally, patients should be hyperoxygenated with 100% oxygen prior to and following suction. (**Ref.** 5, p. 262)

350. D. Ideal suction catheters should incorporate several features to aid in aspiration as well as minimize trauma to the airway. These include:
1. side holes to dissipate the vacuum over a wider surface area and to prevent adherence to the tracheal wall
2. possessing a length of 20 to 22 in. in length to allow the tip of the catheter to pass through the artificial airway
3. having smooth edges to prevent and avoid tracheal damage. (**Ref.** 5, p. 260)

351. D. Lung collapse may occur during suction if the diameter of the catheter exceeds one-half the diameter of the airway. This is caused by the inability to properly move air around the catheter and by the application of suction which would in turn collapse the areas distal to the airway. Arrythmias and hypotension may result secondary to vagal stimulation and/or hypoxia. (**Ref.** 5, p. 259)

352. A. Driving mechanisms provide the force that drives the flow of gas necessary to deliver the volume to the patient. This may be accomplished by the use of pneumatics, electronics, or fluidics. (**Ref.** 22, p. 433)

353. B. A negative pressure ventilator applying a subatmospheric pressure to the thorax, thereby causing a decrease in pressure in the lungs relative to the pressure at the mouth, results in the flow of gas. (**Ref.** 22, p. 433)

354. C. A limit is a physical parameter that prevents either flow, volume, time, or pressure from exceeding a preset setting. It is not a function of the primary cycling mechanism. (**Ref.** 22, p. 438)

355. D. Positive pressure ventilators apply supra-atmospheric pressure to the airway to deliver tidal volumes. (**Ref.** 22, p. 433)

356. E. Powering mechanisms are the physical source that result in the operation of ventilators. They may be electric or pneumatic or a combination of both. (**Ref.** 22, p. 433)

357. A. A sine wave produces a sigmoidal flow pattern by logarithmically accelerating decelerating flow by piston-driven devices. (**Ref.** 22, p. 436)

358. B. Accelerating flow patterns produce nonlinear wave forms through nonconstant flow generators. Flow progressively increases throughout inspiration. (**Ref.** 22, p. 436)

359. C. A square wave gas flow is obtained by ventilating a patient at a constant flow throughout the inspiratory cycle and is said to be rectilinear. (**Ref.** 22, p. 435)

360. D. Decelerating flow patterns form parabolic pressure curves by beginning at maximum flow followed by a decaying flow pattern. (**Ref.** 22, p. 436)

361. D. Ventilators may be powered by several mechanisms. These include an electrical source (normally 120 V) a pneumatic source (usually 40 to 60 psi), or a combination of both. (**Ref.** 22, p. 433)

362. C. The type of driving mechanism in a ventilator and the resistance to gas flow to deliver a consistent gas flow pattern. An example of this would be a piston-driven ventilator that results in a sine wave flow pattern due to its physical characteristic of motion. (**Ref.** 22, p. 434)

363. C. If a ventilator can maintain a driving pressure 5 times higher than the system pressure during a mechanical breath it is said to be a flow generator. This principle holds true even in the face of increasing back pressure. (**Ref.** 22, p. 434)

364. B. Ventilators that cannot exceed system pressures at least 5 times the driving pressures demonstrate large variations in gas flows in the face of back pressure. These are said to be pressure generators. (**Ref.** 22, p. 434)

365. D. Volume, pressure, time, and flow can each be the cycling parameter for mechanical ventilators.
1. Volume once reached may cycle the ventilator off.
2. Pressure exceeding a preset limit could signal the ventilator to terminate flow.
3. If a preset time period for inspiratory is reached, this could be the termination signal.
4. If inspiratory flow decreases to a preset limit, the ventilator could cycle off. (**Ref.** 22, p. 437)

366. C. When the primary cycling parameter is reached gas flow terminates. No alarms are activated, as this is a normal function. Secondary cycling parameters function as alarms and are activated when their limits are exceeded. (**Ref.** 22, p. 437)

367. A. The Bird Mark 7 and Bird Mark 8 both are pressure-cycled ventilators. The Bennett PR series are flow- and time-cycled while the Veriflo CV 2000 is time-cycled. (**Ref.** 44, p. 446)

368. C. *Acinetobacter colcoaceticus* has been found to be a causative agent of pneumonias in Wright Respirometers and Bennett Monitoring Spirometers. This organism is generally found in water and soil, and is seen as a Gram-negative rod. (**Ref.** 36, p. 86)

369. C. Similar to a sneeze, exhaled particles from ventilators can remain airborn as far as 10 ft. (**Ref.** 28, p. 246)

370. B. Multiplying of a patient's minute volume by a factor of 4 to 6 will estimate his/her peak inspiratory flow rate. (**Ref.** 28, p. 263)

371. C. Cascade humidifiers have been named safe in regard to being a bacteria producer. This is due to the fact that they produce a vapor, thus not allowing bacteria to travel upon particulate matter. (**Ref.** 28, p. 243)

372. A. A nebulizer can be responsible for bacterial transport due to the particulate aerosol it produces. The particle size is less than 5μ. (**Ref.** 36, p. 84)

373. A. In the assist control mode the ventilator functions much the same as the assist mode unless the patient's respiratory rate falls below a preset level. At this point, the ventilator will switch into a control mode with a backup rate. (**Ref.** 22, p. 439)

374. B. In a control mode, the ventilator is responsible for the initiation of the breath by a time cycle and also for the delivered tidal volume. (**Ref.** 22, p. 439)

375. C. Intermittent mandatory ventilation allows patients to breathe spontaneously with controlled breaths being delivered at preset intervals similar to the control mode. (**Ref.** 22, p. 439)

376. D. In an assist mode, tidal volume is controlled by the ventilator; however, respiratory rate is entirely dependent upon patient demand. In this mode, should a patient become apneic, ventilation will not be provided by the ventilator. (**Ref.** 22, p. 439)

377. C. In order for pressure support-delivered breaths to terminate, inspiratory flow rates must decrease to approximately 25% of the peak inspiratory flow rate. There often are backup mechanisms to terminate inspiratory flow if this primary mechanism fails. (**Ref.** 22, p. 439)

378. B. SIMV describes a mode where patients are permitted to breathe spontaneously with mechanical breathes being interposed at preset intervals that are synchronized to the patient's inspiratory demands. (**Ref.** 22, p. 439)

379. D. Sighs are set mechanical breaths often 50% greater than tidal volumes designed to prevent atelectasis. Inflation hold originally was incorporated to improve gas distribution, but since has dropped in use due to its negative effects on cardiac output. Flow taper provides operators the option of modifying inspiratory airway maneuvers. (**Ref.** 22, p. 440)

380. D. NEEP (negative end expiratory pressure) theoretically prevents increases in mean intrathoracic pressure; however, is not recommended due to the promotion of air trapping and pulmonary edema. PEEP (positive end expiratory pressure) has been shown to improve oxygenation refractory to high oxygen concentrations. Expiratory retard is used to prevent premature closure of small airways which may lead to air trapping; however, this too may decrease cardiac output. (**Ref.** 22, p. 440)

381. B. Both the Bird Mark 7 and Bennett PR-1 are operated completely by pneumatics. The Bear 1 and Puritan Bennett 7200 both possess pneumatic systems but are powered by electrical systems. (**Ref.** 22, pp. 441, 444, 458)

382. A. Double circuit ventilators describe systems which incorporate one compressed gas source to deliver another gas source. Bennett MA-1's and Engstrom Ericas both utilize this type of system. Emersons and Bear 2's are both single circuit systems. (**Ref.** 18)

383. B. The Emerson 3-PV postoperative ventilator utilizes a piston mechanism to achieve a sine wave flow pattern which produces a sigmoidal pattern on pressure waveforms. (**Ref.** 22, p. 442)

384. D. Both the Bear 1 and MA-2 only offer PEEP as an expiratory maneuver. The MA-1 offers expiratory retard in addition to PEEP. (**Ref.** 22, p. 444)

385. C. Neither the MA-1 nor the Bear 1 have built-in oxygen analyzers. The Servo 900C incorporated a Hi/Lo oxygen alarm direct from the manufacturer. (**Ref.** 22, p. 448)

386. D. In order to prevent baratrauma to patients, the Bear 1 incorporates limits to terminate inspiration for pressure flow and time. Volume indirectly is limited should a high pressure alarm be activated. (**Ref.** 22, p. 445)

387. B. Once activated, the alarm silence on the series of Bear ventilators will remain silenced for a period of 60 sec unless depressed a second time. (**Ref.** 18)

388. B. On the Bear 2 ventilator, if the sensitivity is in the most sensitive position (5 o'clock), the patient must generate a -1.0 cm H_2O at 2 L/min. (**Ref.** 18)

389. A. When supplemental oxygen is dialed in on the Bear 2, the oxygen inlet pressure must be at least 27.5 ± 2.5 psig to prevent an audible/visual low O_2 pressure alarm from being activated. (**Ref.** 18)

390. D. In spontaneous breathing modes, the I:E ratio becomes deactivated on the Bear 2. This is primarily due to the fact that the patient determines I:E ratio based on his/her own inspiratory and expiratory demands. (**Ref.** 18)

391. B. The maximal amount of PEEP obtained on a Bear 1 is 30 cm H_2O when using the integrated PEEP valve. Should greater than 30 cm H_2O be desired, external PEEP may be applied; however, the machine would no longer be PEEP-compensated.

392. B. Since the pressure limits on the Bear 1 and Bear 2 are triggered by the machine pressure; you would expect a pressure alarm to activate at a lower pressure on the proximal airway gauge than what is set as the alert/limit. Generally, a gradient of 5 to 15 cm H_2O exists between machine and proximal pressure. (**Ref.** 18)

393. B. The range of tidal volume on a Bear 1 is 100 to 2000 cc. (**Ref.** 18)

394. C. Since the apnea period on a Bear 1 is preset at 20 sec, the ventilator will alarm if the total rate falls below 3 breaths/min. (**Ref.** 18)

395. D. When the nebulizer on a Bear 1 is activated, the gas source used is taken directly from the delivered tidal volume, thereby having no effect on the delivered volume or oxygen concentration. (**Ref.** 18)

396. A. Assist/control and SIMV modes are spontaneous modes which necessitate compensatory mechanisms for PEEP. Since the control mode essentially locks out spontaneous breaths, PEEP compensation is negated. (**Ref.** 18)

397. B. With the application of PEEP on a Bear I, any drop in pressure, whether caused by a leak or patient demand, will result in flow from the demand valve. This flow may be delivered as high as 100 L/min. (**Ref.** 18)

398. B. As with the Bear 1, if the nebulizer on the MA-1 is activated, gas is taken from the delivered tidal volume to power the nebulizer. This will result in no change to delivered tidal volume or oxygen concentration. (**Ref.** 18)

399. A. When using the PEEP valve attachment for the MA-1 the maximum obtainable PEEP level is 15 cm H_2O. This may be enhanced by the addition of auxiliary PEEP devices. (**Ref.** 18)

400. C. The tidal volume range on the MA-1 ventilator is 0 to 2200 cc. (**Ref.** 18)

401. B. Ventilator rates on the MA-1 are available in a range from 0 to 60 breaths/min. (**Ref.** 18)

402. D. Use of PEEP/CPAP can help maintain lung volumes at more normal levels in the face of lung damage. It reduces intra-pulmonary shunting and hypoxemia by improving ventilation (surface area) for gas to diffuse across. Compliance improves with an inversely proportional decrease in airway resistance. (**Ref.** 45)

403. A. In order to meet the demands of decreased compliance and increased resistance often seen in long-term ventilation, high pressure and high flows should be available to ensure adequate ventilation. (**Ref.** 45)

404. C. Since augmented minute ventilation on the Bear 5 has the capability to be completely spontaneous ventilation, it is not necessary to get a back-up rate when ventilating patients in this mode.

405. A. Rate may be achieved in the 0–150 breaths/min range on the Bear 5 to accommodate both neonates and adults. (**Ref.** 18)

406. C. The maximum sigh volume obtained on the Bear 5 is 3000 cc and usually set as 1 1/2 times the set tidal volume. (**Ref.** 18)

407. D. Peak flows on the Bear 5 can be set between 5 and 10 L/min. Delivered peak flows on patients demand can be achieved up to 170 L/min. (**Ref.** 18)

408. D. In the time cycle mode it is necessary to set a constant flow. Since this is not a spontaneous mode and pressure support is a flow variable modality, these two modes cannot be utilized at the same time. (**Ref.** 18)

409. D. On the Puritan Bennett 7200 the PEEP/CPAP adjustment is the only parameter controlled by a knob. All other parameters are microprocessor-controlled. (**Ref.** 45, p. 85)

410. D. The Puritan Bennett 7200 like many newer microprocessor ventilators, offers the ability to vary flows in order to achieve several flow patterns. These are sine wave, square, and tapered wave forms. (**Ref.** 45, p. 83)

411. C. In order to obtain ventilator circuit compliance, exhaled volume should be collected from an occluded circuit during a mechanical breath with a set pressure limit. The equation is as follows:

$$\text{Lost volume} = \frac{\text{Tidal volume} - \text{Compressed volume}}{\text{Peak airway pressure} - \text{PEEP}}$$

With an exhaled volume of 240 mL at an occlusion pressure of 60 cm H_2O on the result would be X = 240 mL/60 cm H_2O; X = 4 mL/H_2O. (**Ref.** 46, p. 29)

412. C. Since pressure-cycled ventilators result in a variable delivered tidal volume, inversely proportional to pressure, their use is generally limited to intermittent positive pressure breathing treatments. Preterm infants historically are ventilated by time-cycled ventilators, while volume ventilators are used in recovery rooms. (**Ref.** 46, p. 27)

413. C. Because precise control of inspiratory time and I : E ratios is desired in the ventilation of preterm infants, time-cycled, preset pressure style ventilators are the method of choice when ventilating infants. Some advantages over volume ventilators are:
1. Decreased incidence of pulmonary baratrauma secondary to high airway pressures.
2. Less effect of decreased minute volume due to small endotracheal leaks.
3. The inability of volume preset ventilator to sense patient effort at small tidal volumes. (**Ref.** 46, p. 27)

414. D. The Bourns BP200, Sechrist IV-100B, and Healthdyne 105 are all electrically controlled ventilators that also incorporate a pneumatic gas delivery system. All three are time-cycled, pressure-preset type ventilators used in the ventilation of infants. (**Ref.** 22, p. 454)

415. D. Like most infant ventilators, the BP200 only offers the IMV and CPAP modes in ventilatory support. Assist delivery devices often require greater inspiratory movement than those generated by infants. (**Ref.** 22, p. 454)

416. A. Because the BP200 is a constant flow generator, only a square wave and rectilinear pressure pattern can be obtained. Only variable flow devices can obtain accelerating and decelerating flow patterns. (**Ref.** 22, p. 454)

417. A. The maximum flow obtained by the Sechrist IV-100B is 0 to 32 L/min. At the flush setting, flows as high as 40 L/min can be obtained. (**Ref.** 18)

418. C. The inspiratory pressure range of the Sechrist IV-100B is 7 to 70 cm H_2O. (**Ref.** 18)

419. D. The alarm delay time on the Sechrist IV-100B is 3 to 60 sec. The alarm is disabled each time the pressure needle crosses through the low inspiratory pressure settings. (**Ref.** 18)

420. D. The safety pressure pop-off located behind the integral blender on the Sechrist IV-100B can be adjusted by setting a flow of 5 L/min, occluding the patient connection and exhalation port. The set pop-off can be determined by observing the maximum pressure achieved on the manometer. (**Ref.** 18)

421. A. The normal exhalation valve supplied with the Sechrist IV-100B works best at flows of 3 to 12 L/min. High flow settings may cause delivery of inadvertent PEEP. When this occurs, the pediatric exhalation block may be required. (**Ref.** 18)

422. A. The maximum flow delivery from the Sechrist IV-100B is 40 L/min. At flows this high, use of the pediatric exhalation block may be required to offset flow-induced inadvertent PEEP. (**Ref.** 18)

423. C. When ventilating on infants with a Sechrist IV-100B, the manufacturer recommends setting the low inspiratory pressure alarm approximately 1 to 2 cm H_2O below the maximum airway pressure. (**Ref.** 18)

424. D. All of the above. Flow will determine the slope of the curve during inspiration, inspiratory time will affect the area underneath the curve, while the pressure limit will determine the height of the curve. (**Ref.** 18)

425. A. The minimum expiration time on a Healthdyne 100 ventilator is 0.5 sec with a minimum inspiratory time of 0.1 sec, or a total cycle time of 0.6 sec. Therefore, the maximum rate obtained 100.

426. B. According to manufacturer's specifications, the minimum expiratory time is 0.5 sec.

427. A. The manufacturer-recommended PEEP control is adjustable from 0 to 20 cm H_2O.

428. C. The internal pressure limit control is adjustable from 1 to 50 cm H_2O by manufacturer's specifications.

429. B. The Bio-Med MVP-10 ventilator, popular as an infant transport device, can achieve tidal volumes of 400 mL, dependent upon the delivered flow and inspiratory time. (**Ref.** 18)

430. C. The respiratory rate on the MVP-10 is variable from 0 to 120 breaths/min with inspiratory and expiratory times of 0.25 sec. (Insp) 0.25 sec + (Exp) 0.25 sec = 0.5 sec cycle time. 60 sec/min divided by 0.5 sec = 120 breaths/min. (**Ref.** 18)

431. B. A one-way valve installed at the patient connection of the MVP-10 is designed to open if system pressure falls below -4 cm H_2O during patient inspiration. This safety device allows for patient inspiration in the unlikely event of no gas supply. (**Ref.** 18)

432. A. When using the MVP-10 transport ventilator in nonpressurized aircraft, the inspiratory and expiratory time controls must be corrected to read 2 1/2 times greater than what is set for every 1000 ft above sea level. (**Ref.** 18)

433. B. High-Frequency Ventilation encompasses many forms including High-Frequency Positive-Pressure Ventilation (HFPPV), High-Frequency Jet Ventilation (HFJV) and High-Frequency Oscillation (HFO). In these methods, ventilation is maintained at volumes smaller than anatomical deadspace and at lower airway pressures. Frequency during oscillation may approach 3000 breaths/min. (**Ref.** 18, p. 92)

434. D. High-frequency ventilation due to low tidal volumes and decreased airway pressures may reduce the incidence of pulmonary baratrauma. With the associated decrease, intrathoracic pressure as compared to conventional ventilation, cardiovascular depression is minimized. Mechanical deadspace is unaffected and inherent to all ventilation circuits despite what method of ventilation is chosen. (**Ref.** 48, p. 92)

435. D. Theories as to the mechanism of gas transport with high-frequency ventilation include:
1. Brownian motion, or the intermingling of two gases through diffusion;
2. convection, or the principle of bulk flow as in conventional alveolar ventilation; and
3. augmented transport, which is the combined effect of diffusion and convection. (**Ref.** 48, p. 92)

436. A. At frequencies of 60 to 90 breaths/min, volumes of 200 to 300 cc are achieved. This mode of ventilation is termed High-Frequency Positive-Pressure Ventilation (HFPPV). Airway pressures of 5 to 15 cm H_2O are generally seen. (**Ref.** 48, p. 92)

437. C. Respiratory rates of 100 to 900 breaths/min are utilized in High-Frequency Jet Ventilation (HFJV). Delivered tidal volume ranges from 80 to 140 mL, dependent upon airway compliance. (**Ref.** 48, p. 92)

438. A. Optimal ventilator settings when using High-Frequency Positive-Pressure Ventilation (HFPPV) include 60 breaths/min, with an inspiratory time of 22%. (**Ref.** 12, p. 92)

439. C. Complications associated with High-Frequency Jet Ventilation include:

1. inadequate humidification which could lead to airway occlusion; and

2. damage to the tracheal mucosa secondary to number 1, as well as to the effects of high-velocity gases impacting against airway tissue. HFJV is often used for the treatment of bronchopleural fistulas and pneumothoraxes when conventional ventilation fails. (**Ref.** 48, p. 92)

440. B. When humidification is accomplished by the direct infusion of water into the jet stream, rates of 20 to 30 mL/hr are recommended. Care must be taken not to underinfuse, which could lead to inspissation of secretions; or overinfusion, which could lead to fluid overload. (**Ref.** 48, p. 94)

441. D. High-Frequency Oscillation is accomplished through the use of a piston pump. Rates of 900 to 3000 breaths/min have been successfully used to ventilate most patients. HFO is often expressed as Hertz instead of breaths/min, in which the delivered range would be 15 Hz (000 breaths/min) to 50 Hz (3000 breaths/min). (**Ref.** 48, p. 94)

442. B. Delivered tidal volume during high-frequency oscillating have been estimated at 5 to 80 mL per breath. (**Ref.** 48, p. 94)

443. C. When ventilating with High-Frequency Jet Ventilation, increasing respiratory rate while maintaining a constant % TI will result in increasing the arterial P_{CO_2}. This is due to a decrease in delivered tidal volume. (**Ref.** 55, p. 68)

444. B. Inadvertent PEEP may occur with High-Frequency Ventilation with elevated rates and inspiratory times, which will in effect impinge on expiratory time. If expiratory time is decreased in a diseased lung, air trapping will occur, resulting in inadvertent PEEP with depression of cardiac output. (**Ref.** 48, p. 95)

445. C. Noninvasive support devices for ventilation include Pulmo-wraps, rocking beds, and chest cuirasses. Each has been used primarily for the treatment of patients with neuromusculoskeletal disorders. The LP-6 is a positive-pressure ventilator requiring tracheal intubation. (**Ref.** 50, p. 140)

446. A. The LP-3, LP-4, LP-5, and Thompson M25B are generally all used in home care situations. Of the four listed, the LP-3 has a fixed I : E ratio of 1 : 12, thereby limiting the flow rates delivered to patients. (**Ref.** 50, p. 141)

447. C. In the event of an emergency to a patient at home treated with mechanical ventilation, an air compressor for aerosal medications, a manual resuscitator, and a suction machine should all be available to the patient and/or care givers. Heart monitors are not necessary as pulses are easily palpable. (**Ref.** 50, p. 141)

448. D. For safety purposes, several parameters should be constantly monitored when ventilating patients. The electronic and pneumatic sources provide the mechanism to ventilate the patient. If either source fails, ventilation would be terminated. The fraction of inspired oxygen plays an integral part in assuring adequate cellular homeostasis. Gas temperature should be monitored in order to humidify the delivered gas as well as prevent scalding of the airway. Finally, respiratory rate is a prime indication of a patient's ventilatory status as well as an indication of acid-base status. (**Ref.** 51, p. 135)

449. B. If an electrical failure should occur when ventilating a patient an audible alarm triggered by battery packs should be available and produce an audible tone for at least 5 min. (**Ref.** 51, p. 136)

450. C. Gas source alarms which are incorporated on most ventilators indicate insufficient oxygen pressure when activated. They do not function as an analyzer and will not alarm if the wrong gas type provides the source pressure. (**Ref.** 51, p. 136)

451. A. Polarographic or Clark electrodes are utilized for the determination of FIO_2. Changes in FIO_2 result in an increase or decrease in released electrons from an electrolyte solution. The Severinghaus electrode is used to determine $PaCO_2$. (**Ref.** 51, p. 136)

452. B. When using an oxygen analyzer continuously, calibration should be performed at least every 12 hr. If only used in intervals, calibration needs to be done with each measurement. (**Ref.** 51, p. 137)

453. C. When a polarographic oxygen analyzer is calibrated to ambient pressure then placed on a ventilator, it will indicate a higher than actual FIO_2. This is due to the pressure forcing a greater number of oxygen molecules into the cell. (**Ref.** 51, p. 137)

454. A. When exposed to pressure, a polarographic oxygen analyzer will read 1% higher for each 10 cm H_2O pressure above an atmospheric pressure. (**Ref.** 51, p. 137)

455. C. If a polarographic analyzer is calibrated at zero humidity and then placed in a humidified environment, the displayed concentration will read lower than actual. (**Ref.** 51, p. 137)

456. D. A polarographic analyzer if calibrated to zero humidity when placed in a humidified environment will display 4% less than actual. (**Ref.** 51, p. 137)

457. B. Capnometers determine CO_2 levels through the use of an infrared analyzer by the specific absorption of the CO_2 molecules. The Clark electrode is used for oxygen measurement while the Severinghaus principle is used for CO_2 determination in blood. (**Ref.** 51, p. 138)

458. C. Mass spectrometers can be used to measure respiratory gases. They operate by ionizing a gas sample, then separating the ion particles by their charge. Each gas type has a separate mass-to-charge ratio to distinguish it from other gases. (**Ref.** 51, p. 137)

459. D. Within a carbon dioxide wave form, phase 1 represents deadspace ventilation. It is the initial part of expiration and normally contains no CO_2. (**Ref.** 51, p. 138)

460. A. Phase 2 of a capnogram represents a mixture of deadspace and gas from lung units participating in gas exchange. (**Ref.** 51, p. 138)

461. C. Phase 3 of a capnogram is distinguished by a plateau and represents "alveolar" CO_2 concentration. The peak end expiratory CO_2 concentration approximates the arterial CO_2. (**Ref.** 51, p. 138)

462. C. Normally the peak expired CO_2 is 1 to 7 mmHg lower than the arterial CO_2. In certain disease states, this gradient will be increased even more. (**Ref.** 51, p. 138)

463. B. Sampling ports of CO_2 gas analyzers must be placed between the patient airway and the breathing circuit. If it is placed on the expiratory side it will underestimate the end-tidal CO_2. If placed before the humidification device only inspiratory CO_2 will be reported. (**Ref.** 51, p. 138)

464. C. A plateau on a capnogram represents end-expiration and respiratory pause. It also reflects "alveolar" CO_2 concentration. (**Ref.** 52, p. 13)

465. C. When using transcutaneous oxygen monitors, the electrode must be allowed to stabilize for approximately 30 min before clinical use. This is to allow for warming of the site, and equilibrium of perfusion. (**Ref.** 52, p. 12)

466. D. The $PtcO_2$ reading usually is lower than arterial PO_2; however, it is not equivalent. Although it correlates well with arterial PO_2, certain factors do impair its accuracy. These include hypotension, obesity, acidosis, and anesthetics. (**Ref.** 52, p. 12)

467. B. Electrode placement of transcutaneous oxygen monitors should be rotated every 2 to 4 hr to prevent minor skin burns. (**Ref.** 52, p. 12)

468. D. Hypotension, obesity, acidosis, and certain anesthetics can impair the accuracy of PCO_2 monitors. (**Ref.** 52, p. 12)

469. A. Because pulse oximetry only reflects the saturation of functional hemoglobin, dyshemoglobins such as carboxyhemoglobin and methmeglobin, if present, will not be factored into the oximeter output, thereby possibly causing an overestimation in actual oxygen saturation. This is especially true for smokers and individuals exposed to smoke inhalation, such as fire victims. (**Ref.** 52, p. 12).

470. A. The principal function of aerosol tents is to provide an atmosphere saturated with water that is cooled to provide an environment that promotes a decrease in swelling associated with croup/epiglottitis. It does not necessarily need to provide oxygen and is rarely used in the treatment of asthma. (**Ref.** 18)

471. B. The Ohio Pediatric Aerosol Tent, when placed in the cool mode, will lower the temperature by 6 to 15°F. This is dependent upon the flow output and the size of the individual within the canopy. (**Ref.** 18)

472. B. The Ohio High-Output Pneumatic Nebulizer supplies approximately 4 cc/min. This is similar to the output of an ultrasonic nebulizer. (**Ref.** 18)

473. B. To avoid excess buildup of carbon dioxide within an aerosol tent, the flow should never fall below 10 L/min. If necessary a flap may be cut in the top of the canopy to allow for the release of excess CO_2. (**Ref.** 20)

474. A. The child and infant Laerdal resuscitator incorporates a pressure relief mechanism which is preset at 40 cm H_2O. This device is intended to prevent baratrauma associated with high peak airway pressures. (**Ref.** 18)

475. B. The Puritan PMR2 resuscitator has a reset safety valve on all units that are preset to pop off at 45 cm H_2O pressure. (**Ref.** 18)

476. D. With a Laerdal resuscitator, an FIO_2 of 1.00 can be obtained with the adult bag when using a reservoir at volumes below 750 mL, rates less than 12, and oxygen flow rates greater than 12 L/min. When using the child resuscitation unit, an FIO_2 of 1.00 can be obtained when using the reservoir bag and an oxygen flow rate of 1 times minute ventilation volume.

477. C. According to manufacturer's specifications, the volume of the Laerdal adult resuscitator bag is 1600 mL.

478. B. According to manufacturer's specifications, the volume is 500 mL.

479. C. According to manufacturer's specifications, the volume is 240 mL.

480. A. According to manufacturer's specifications, the oxygen reservoir bag capacity used on both the adult and child resuscitator is 2600 mL.

481. C. According to manufacturer's specifications, the oxygen reservoir bag for the infant resuscitator has a capacity of 600 mL.

482. C. Endotracheal tubes are hollow airways shaped to fit the natural curvature of the upper respiratory tract. They vary in length from 12 cm (neonate) to 38 cm (adult). (**Ref.** 60, p. 170)

483. A. The internal diameter of endotracheal tubes ranges from 2.5 mm in neonates to 11 mm in adults. When suctioning from these airways, the lumen of the catheter should not exceed one-half of the internal diameter of the endotracheal tube. (**Ref.** 60, p. 170)

484. D. The endotracheal tubes are made of several materials, including rubber, silicon, nylon, and teflon. The most common used material is PVC (polyvinyl chloride). These materials are nontoxic and nonreactive so as to prevent an inflammatory response by their insertion. (**Ref.** 60, p. 170)

485. C. All tubes used in airway management must meet the federal standards of implantation testing for toxicity and tissue reactivity set forth by the Z-79 committee. Those tubes passing will be marked by Z-79 or IT. Tubes should also be labeled by internal diameter and tubing length. The external diameter should also be included. The type of cuff may be high- or low-pressure, but is not delineated on the tube. (**Ref.** 60, p. 171)

486. C. The IT on endotracheal tubes stands for implantation testing for toxicity and tissue reactivity. These standards are set forth by the committee on anesthesia equipment of the U.S.A. Standards Institute. (**Ref.** 60, p. 170)

487. B. The preferred cuff on a tracheal device is one of high-volume, low-pressure balloon to lessen the possibilities of tracheal malascia. (**Ref.** 60, p. 171)

488. D. The curved blade on a laryngoscope may also be referred to as a MacIntosh blade. It is used by inserting it into the valacula, lifting and moving the epiglottis away from the vocal cords. (**Ref.** 60, p. 171)

489. A. The straight blade of a laryngoscope may also be referred to as a Miller blade. It is used to directly move the epiglottis from the vocal cords. (**Ref.** 60, p. 172)

490. C. A long-nosed forceps may be used during intubation to guide a nasotracheal tube into the trachea. It may also be used in endotracheal intubation if the stylet is unavailable. (**Ref.** 60, p. 173)

491. B. When using a stylet for endotracheal intubation, the distal end of the rod should be ½ in. from the end of the tube. This prevents tracheal damage by the stylet. (**Ref.** 60, p. 172)

492. B. Tracheal capillary blood pressure is approximately 25 mmHg. Therefore, cuff pressures should not exceed this level or the patient is at increased risk of tissue necrosis. (**Ref.** 60, p. 174)

493. D. Cuff inflation pressure should be checked at least once every 8 hr, or at each time the cuff is inflated. (**Ref.** 60, p. 175)

494. B. Tracheostomy tubes may vary in length from 2 to 6 in. and may be designed with or without a cuff. (**Ref.** 60, p. 173)

495. A. Tracheostomy tubes are designed with an internal diameter ranging from 2 to 22 mm. Their material is similar to that of an endotracheal tube. (**Ref.** 60, p. 175)

496. C. Permanent tracheostomy tubes are made out of silver because this substance is nontoxic and does not react to tissue. (**Ref.** 60, p. 175)

497. D. Tracheostomy buttons are used to maintain stoma patency by preventing it from closing. Conversely they are also used in the process of weaning a patient by allowing gradual stoma closure. (**Ref.** 60, p. 176)

498. C. Without an artificial airway in place, the tracheostomy would close within 48 to 72 hr. (**Ref.** 60, p. 177)

499. B. The inner cannula of a tracheostomy tube should be cleaned at least every 8 hr utilizing 2% hydrogen peroxide, or more often as necessary. (**Ref.** 60, p. 179)

500. C. The inner cannula is cleaned using 2% hydrogen peroxide. Soaps or Cidex should not be used because of the chance of residue being left in the tube. (**Ref.** 60, p. 179)

501. A. When performing intubation, the laryngoscope is used in the left hand. This is necessary because the design of the blades require intubation on the right side relative to the person performing intubation. Otherwise, if holding the laryngoscope with the right hand, you would obstruct the view of the trachea. (**Ref.** 60, p. 180)

502. C. The safe therapeutic range for aspiration in the pediatric patient is between 80 and 100 mmHg. An adult may be suctioned at pressures between 120 and 150 mmHg. (**Ref.** 60, p. 196)

503. B. The safe therapeutic range for endotracheal suction in the neonate is 60 to 80 mmHg. (**Ref.** 60, p. 197)

504. B. The connecting tubing in reservoir jars from the vacuum equipment should be changed every 48 hr to inhibit bacterial growth. (**Ref.** 60, p. 197)

505. A. For endotracheal suctioning the patient should be placed in a semi-Fowler's position. This will facilitate greater patency. (**Ref.** 60, p. 201)

506. C. Prior to suctioning, a patient receiving oxygen should be administered 100% oxygen for 1 min prior to suctioning. This helps to prevent hypoxemia and atelectasis. (**Ref.** 60, p. 201)

507. B. Suction should not be applied continuously, but intermittently upon withdrawal. This would prevent the catheter from adhering to the tracheal wall. The catheter should be advanced as far as possible and rotated 360 deg. upon withdrawal. The procedure should not take more than 20 sec. (**Ref.** 60, p. 206)

508. A. The FIO_2 possible in an oxygen tent is approximately 30% to 50% at flows of 10 to 15 L/min. (**Ref.** 60, p. 24)

509. D. The FIO_2 obtained in an oxygen hood can be as high as 100% due to the size in relation to the size of the patient. (**Ref.** 60, p. 24)

510. B. The Wheatstone Bridge principle of oxygen analyzing is the same as thermal conductivity. This describes the way the gas conducts heat. A change in gas concentration will result in a change in conductivity. This will cause a change — resistance thereby indication the change in oxygen concentration. (**Ref.** 60, p. 35)

511. A. The particle size generated by the SPAG-2 is 95% less than 5 μ in diameter. (**Ref.** 18)

512. C. When preparing virazole, the drug is packaged in a lyphosized (powdered) form. Therefore, 300 mL of sterile water must be mixed to produce an aqueous solution. (**Ref.** 18)

513. A. The SPAG-2 requires an operational pressure of 26 psig. (**Ref.** 18)

514. C. The flow rate output of a SPAG-2 generator is 12.5 to 15 L/min. (**Ref.** 18)

515. B. Virazole, which is an aqueous solution, may be stored at room temperature and at sterile condition for up to 24 hr. (**Ref.** 18)

516. B. A virazole solution still under use for longer than 24 hr should be replaced with a new solution. (**Ref.** 18)

517. A. The administration of virazole may be carried out for 12 to 18 hr/day for a minimum of 3 days depending on the severity of the disease. Treatment should be instituted as soon as possible unless RSV is suspected. (**Ref.** 18)

518. B. Recommended delivery device for virazole is through an oxygen hood. Presently, scavenger mechanisms are being developed to prevent exposure to health care personnel. Virazole should not be used with ventilators due to the possibilities of expiratory occlusion. Virazole should also not be used with oxygen tents because the humidity will alter the particle size, thereby changing the site of deposition. (**Ref.** 18)

519. B. Virazole should not be administered for more than 7 days. (**Ref.** 18)

9 Pathophysiology

DIRECTIONS (Questions 520–600): Each of the questions or incomplete statements below is followed by four suggested answers or completions. Select the **one** that is **best** in each case.

520. In which age group(s) does the highest mortality occur with influenza?
1. 5 to 9 years
2. 25 to 35 years
3. Infancy
4. Over age 50
   A. 4. only
   B. 3. only
   C. 3. and 4.
   D. None of the above

521. Which of the following groups should be vaccinated and kept immunized by annual booster injections for influenza?
1. Chronic cardiac
2. Chronic respiratory
3. Diabetes
4. Infancy
   A. 1. and 2.
   B. 1., 2., and 3.
   C. 1., 2., and 4.
   D. All of the above

522. Which of the following organisms are most commonly isolated from the secretions in chronic bronchitis?
    1. Klebsiella
    2. Staphylococci
    3. Streptococci
    4. Pneumococci
       A. 2. and 3.
       B. 1. only
       C. 1., 2., 3., and 4.
       D. 4. only

523. A persistant cough in which more than 1 oz of sputum is raised in a day is an essential feature of which of the following?
    A. Bronchitis
    B. Influenza
    C. Common cold
    D. Pneumonia

524. Bronchiectasis is caused by
    A. chronic bronchitis
    B. bronchial obstruction
    C. chronic sinusitis
    D. none of the above

525. Which of the following types of bronchial dilatation are seen with bronchiectasis?
    A. Cylindrical
    B. Saccular
    C. Fusiform
    D. All of the above

526. Which of the following is the primary causative agent of bacterial pneumonia?
    A. Pneumococcus
    B. Streptococcus
    C. Klebsiella
    D. Staphylococcus

527. *Klebsiella* sputum has which of the following characteristic colors?
   A. Rust
   B. Gray
   C. Cherry red
   D. Yellow

528. Which of the following is the most useful aid in following the clinical course of bacterial pneumonia?
   A. Chest x-ray
   B. Blood culture
   C. Leukocyte count
   D. Erythrocyte count

529. Which of the following is incorrect about bronchiectasis?
   A. Has no damaging effect socially
   B. Chief symptoms are cough, sputum production, and blood spitting
   C. Two or more lobes often are involved
   D. Moist rales over the base of the lungs

530. Which of the following organisms cause almost all pulmonary tuberculosis in humans?
   A. *Mycobacterium bovis*
   B. *Mycobacterium tuberculosis*
   C. *Mycobacterium avis*
   D. *Mycobacterium fortuitum*

531. Pulmonary tuberculosis almost always occurs in which area of the lungs?
   1. Upper part
   2. Lower part
   3. Apex of one lung
   4. Right lung
   5. Left lung
      A. 2. and 5.
      B. 1. and 3.
      C. 1., 3., and 4.
      D. 1. and 4.

532. Tuberculosis may be spread
  1. in the lung by direct extension in the involved lobe
  2. by the lymphatics to other parts of the body
  3. by the bloodstream, if a caseous focus erodes into a vein
  4. by going through the eustachian tubes
    A. 1., 2., and 3.
    B. 3. only
    C. 1. and 3.
    D. all of the above

533. Which of the following is true of tuberculous pneumonia?
    A. Profound toxemia
    B. Extensive death of lung tissue
    C. None of the above
    D. Both A. and B.

534. Which of the following groups are more often victims of tuberculosis?
  1. Infants and children under age 15
  2. Black women early age
  3. White women any age
  4. Black men between 45 and 64 years of age.
  5. White men between 45 and 64 years of age
    A. 4. only
    B. 2., 4., and 5.
    C. 2. and 4.
    D. All of the above

535. Which of the following methods is the most accurate for discovering early pulmonary tuberculosis?
    A. Physical signs
    B. Tuberculin skin test
    C. Chest x-ray
    D. Sputum examination

536. Which of the following is not a tuberculin skin test?
    A. Mantoux test
    B. Papanicolaou test
    C. Heaf test
    D. Mono-Vacc test

537. Which of the following is INCORRECT about histoplasmosis?
   A. There is direct infection from person to person
   B. *Histoplasma capsulatum* grows in the soil and bears spores called sycelial phase
   C. Yeast phase grows in the body to produce the disease
   D. People inhaling spores in dust develop the disease

538. When histoplasmosis is present with obscure fever, which organ will show enlargement?
   1. Heart
   2. Liver
   3. Spleen
   4. Pancreas
      A. 2. and 3.
      B. 2., 3., and 4.
      C. 3. and 4.
      D. All of the above

539. Which of the following diseases is treated with isoniazid?
   A. Histoplasmosis
   B. Mycoplasma pneumonia
   C. Bronchiectasis
   D. Tuberculosis

540. Which of the following diseases is caused by inhaling infected dust containing spores?
   1. Histoplasmosis
   2. Coccidiodommycosis
   3. Blastomycosis
   4. Myocardiosis
      A. 1. and 2.
      B. 1., 2., and 3.
      C. 3. and 4.
      D. All of the above

541. On auscultation of the chest, musical sounds ranging from course wheezes to a high-pitched piping over both lungs are observed with
A. bronchitis
B. asthma
C. pneumonia
D. bronchiectasis

542. What method is used to determine degrees of functional impairment due to emphysema?
A. Measuring lung ventilation
B. Measuring lung volumes
C. Measuring gas exchange
D. All of the above

543. Which type of emphysema causes scarring in the lungs?
A. Primary
B. Bullous
C. Paracicatarical
D. None of the above

544. What percentage of emphysematous patients were heavy smokers?
A. 50%
B. 70%
C. 80%
D. More than 90%

545. Polycythemia is present in which of the following?
A. Bronchectasis
B. Emphysema
C. Asthma
D. Bronchitis

546. In the final stage of emphysema, the overloaded heart reaches its limit of muscular compensation and begins to fail (cor pulmonale). Which of the following symptoms occur?
1. Destruction of a large part of the capillaries in the lungs
2. Lower blood oxygen
3. Shunting of unaerated blood
4. Overworking the right ventricle
    A. 1. only
    B. 2. and 4.
    C. 1., 2., and 3.
    D. All of the above

547. A battery of physiological tests and formulas has been developed to diagnose emphysema. Which of the following establish the stages of the disease?
    A. Forced expiratory volume
    B. Oxygen and carbon dioxide content of arterial blood
    C. The pH content of arterial blood
    D. All of the above

548. Obstructions to the smaller air passages are relieved by
    A. treating the infection
    B. thinning secretions by increase in fluid intake, expectorants, and humidifying or wetting agents
    C. giving drugs that will dilate the bronchi
    D. all of the above

549. Which of the following bronchogenic carcinomas occurs most frequently?
    A. Undifferentiated carcinoma
    B. Oat cell carcinoma
    C. Squamous cell carcinoma
    D. Adrenocarcinoma

550. A solitary nodule ("corn lesion") in the peripheral portion of the lung is the most typical early x-ray finding in
    A. bronchogenic carcinoma
    B. tuberculosis
    C. emphysema
    D. asthma

551. Patients with V/Q abnormalities and intrapulmonary shunting require
    A. control ventilation
    B. assisted ventilation
    C. SIMV
    D. CPAP

552. In severe cases of ARDS, what is necessary to effect adequate ventilation?
    1. High peak inflation pressures
    2. Large tidal volumes
    3. Low peak inflation pressures
    4. Small tidal volumes
        A. 1. only
        B. 1. and 2.
        C. 3. and 4.
        D. 2. only

553. High-Frequency Ventilation (HFV) has been particularly useful in
    A. bronchopleural fistula
    B. refractory cases of hyaline membrane disease
    C. newborn diaphragmatic hernia
    D. all of the above

554. Which of the following is not a cardiovascular complication associated with mechanical ventilation?
    A. Increased cardiac output
    B. Altered cerebral blood flow, intracranial pressure
    C. V/Q abnormalities
    D. All of the above

555. Which of the following is a pulmonary complication associated with mechanical ventilation?
    1. Pneumothorax
    2. Subcutaneous emphysema
    3. Vascular air embolization
    4. Pneumomediastinum
        A. 1. and 2.
        B. 1., 2., and 3.
        C. None of the above
        D. All of the above

556. In severe cases of respiratory distress, oxygen consumption associated with spontaneous breathing may be as much as what percent of total body oxygen consumption?
   A. 40%
   B. 25%
   C. 30%
   D. 20%

557. Once a mode of volume ventilation is selected, specific ventilator parameters must be determined to effect the desired physiological response in the patient. Which of the following are independent variables that must be accounted for?
   1. Tidal volume (TV)
   2. Respiratory rate (RR)
   3. Flow rate (V)
   4. Inspiratory/expiratory ratio (I:E)
   5. Oxygen concentration (FIO_2)
   6. Positive end-expiratory pressure (PEEP)
      A. All but 6.
      B. 1., 2., and 3.
      C. All of the above
      D. 1., 2., 3., and 5.

558. In a patient who is not breathing spontaneously, what ventilatory rates are usually sufficient to maintain adequate alveolar ventilation?
   A. 10 to 14 breaths/min
   B. 8 to 12 breaths/min
   C. 12 to 16 breaths/min
   D. 18 to 20 breaths/min

559. Patients whose lung disease is characterized by impaired expiratory flows may need an inspiratory/expiratory (I:E) ratio of
   A. 1:2
   B. 1:3
   C. 1:4 or greater
   D. none of the above

560. Compressible volume should always be accounted for in volume ventilation of small children because what percent of delivered volume can be "lost" to ventilator circuits?
  A. 20%
  B. 50%
  C. 70%
  D. 80%

561. During volume ventilation it is common to use a tidal volume of
  A. 10 to 15 mL/kg
  B. 7 to 10 mL/kg
  C. 5 to 7 mL/kg
  D. 16 to 18 mL/kg

562. The rate of gas flow delivered by the ventilator should be selected to conform to which of the following criteria?
  A. Patient comfort
  B. Low airway turbulence
  C. Sufficient time for pulmonary emptying
  D. All of the above

563. In which of the following is HFV used postoperatively?
  1. Laryngoscopy
  2. Bronchoscopy
  3. Thoracotomies
  4. Neurosurgery
     A. 1. and 2.
     B. 3. only
     C. All but 4.
     D. All of the above

564. Both shock and respiratory failure can result from which of the common etiologic factors?
  A. Hemorrhagic pancreatitis
  B. Aspiration of gastric contents
  C. Fat emboli
  D. All of the above

565. Which of the following is the measurement of intravascular volume?
A. Pulmonary arterial pressure
B. Wedge pressure
C. Arterial pressure
D. Central venous pressure

566. Which of the following is a means to assess left ventricular function?
A. Pulmonary arterial and wedge pressure
B. Arterial pressure
C. Central venous pressure
D. None of the above

567. Which of the following is an indication for emergency tracheostomy?
1. Severe facial fractures
2. Massive intraoral bleeding
3. Laryngotracheal injury
4. Cervical spine injury
    A. 1., 2., and 3.
    B. 1. and 2.
    C. 2. and 3.
    D. All of the above

568. Which of the following indicates a "flail segment"?
A. Single rib fractured in two places
B. Multiple fractured ribs
C. Bilateral fractured ribs
D. None of the above

569. Increases in $PeCO_2$ may be caused by
1. Hypoventilation
2. Increased CO
3. Hyperthermia
4. Rebreathing
    A. 1. and 4.
    B. 1., 2., and 3.
    C. 1., 2., and 4.
    D. All of the above

570. Decreases in $PeCO_2$ may be caused by
    1. hyperventilation
    2. apnea
    3. reduced cardiac output
    4. hyperthermia
        A. 1. and 3.
        B. 1., 2., and 4.
        C. 1., 2., and 3.
        D. All of the above

571. Effort to create negative pressure equal and opposite to the sum of PEEP and the opening pressure valve
    1. increases work of breathing
    2. decreases work of breathing
    3. augments venous return to right heart and increases stroke volume
    4. may increase cardiac output
        A. 1. only
        B. 1., 3., and 4.
        C. 2., 3., and 4.
        D. none of the above

572. Patients that are at significant risk of developing postoperative pulmonary complications are
    A. those having a forced vital capacity (FVC) less than 70% of predicted
    B. those having a ratio of forced expiratory volume for 1 sec to FVC (FEV_1/FVC) less than 65%
    C. both A. and B.
    D. none of the above

573. Oxygen toxicity is likely to occur if there is prolonged exposure to
    A. FIO_2 1.0 at 1ALA
    B. FIO_2 0.5 at 1ALA
    C. FIO_2 0.6 at 1ALA
    D. none of the above

574. What percent of AIDS patients have involvement of the lungs?
   A. 40%
   B. 50%
   C. 60%
   D. 70%

575. Which of the following is a noninfectious pulmonary complication of AIDS?
   A. Karposi's sarcoma
   B. *Pneumocystis carinii*
   C. cytomegalovirus

576. To provide accurate results when obtaining mixed venous oxygen saturation samples (SvO_2), blood should be drawn
   A. from the pulmonary artery
   B. from the pulmonary vein.
   C. quickly to prevent clotting within the catheter.
   D. slowly to prevent arterial admixture.
   E. both A. and C.

577. Pulmonary artery diastolic pressures may be used to estimate pulmonary artery wedge pressures in the absence of
   A. mitral stenosis
   B. pulmonary emboli
   C. tachycardia
   D. both A. and B.
   E. all of the above

578. Which of the following is necessary for diagnosing Karposi's sarcoma?
   A. Gallium scan
   B. Fiberoptic bronchoscopy
   C. Open lung biopsy
   D. None of the above

579. The peak incidence of pulmonary fat embolism syndrome is
   A. 24 hr
   B. 2 to 3 days
   C. 12 hr
   D. 5 to 7 days

580. Situations decreasing the effectiveness of the cough include
   A. central nervous system depression
   B. placement of endotracheal tube
   C. disease conditions in which the patient becomes weak and debilitated
   D. all of the above

581. High-risk factors for nosocomial infections include which of the following?
   1. Chronic debilitation and malnourishment
   2. Underlying chronic pulmonary disease
   3. Extensive tissue trauma
   4. Immunosuppressive agents
      A. 1. and 2.
      B. 1., 2., and 4.
      C. 2. and 3.
      D. All of the above

582. Following intubation, colonization of the respiratory tract by Gram-negative microbes occurs within
   A. 72 hr
   B. 48 hr
   C. 24 hr
   D. 8 hr

583. Oxygen therapy offers little benefit to which of the following?
   1. Hypoventilation
   2. Diffusion impairments
   3. Right-to-left shunts
   4. Ventilation perfusion mismatch
      A. 1. and 2.
      B. 3. only
      C. 1. and 3.
      D. None of the above

584. Indications for use of artificial airways include
1. to prevent or relieve upper airway obstruction
2. to protect airway from aspiration
3. to facilitate tracheal suction
4. to provide a sealed, closed system for mechanical ventilation or CPAP
   - **A.** 3. and 4.
   - **B.** 1., 3., and 4.
   - **C.** 2. and 4.
   - **D.** all of the above

585. Which of the following are adverse reactions with the administration of virazole (ribavirin)?
1. Worsening of respiratory status
2. Pneumothorax
3. Apnea
4. Ventilator dependence
5. Hypotension
   - **A.** 1., 2., and 5.
   - **B.** 2., 3., and 4.
   - **C.** 5. only
   - **D.** All of the above

586. Which of the following are predisposing factors to pulmonary embolism?
1. Advanced age
2. Bed rest
3. Obesity
4. Cardiac arrhythmia
5. Smoking
   - **A.** 2., 3., and 4.
   - **B.** 2. only
   - **C.** 1., 2., and 3.
   - **D.** All of the above

587. The most common symptom of pulmonary embolic disease is
- **A.** dyspnea
- **B.** pleural pain
- **C.** hemotysis
- **D.** sweating

588. The most common physical finding of pulmonary embolic disease is
- **A.** rales
- **B.** tachypnea
- **C.** tachycardia
- **D.** friction rub

589. Most patients with pulmonary embolic disease will have arterial blood gases which present
- **A.** acute respiratory acidosis and hypoxemia
- **B.** acute respiratory alkalosis and hypoxemia
- **C.** acute metabolic acidosis
- **D.** acute metabolic alkalosis

590. Alpha-antitrypsin deficiency may lead to
- **A.** asthma
- **B.** pneumonitis
- **C.** COPD
- **D.** lung cancer

591. The normal serum alpha-antitrypsin is
- **A.** 120 to 150 mg/dL
- **B.** 180 to 244 mg/dL
- **C.** 220 to 280 mg/dL
- **D.** 250 to 320 mg/dL

592. The first pulmonary function test value to become abnormal in COPD is
- **A.** FEV_1
- **B.** MVV
- **C.** FEVC
- **D.** FEF 25% to 75%

593. Which of the following pulmonary function values tends to remain normal until COPD is moderately advanced?
- **A.** FEV_1
- **B.** MVV
- **C.** FEVC
- **D.** FEF 25% to 75%

594. Which of the following lung volumes are increased with COPD?
1. RV
2. VC
3. TLC
4. IRV
    A. 1. only
    B. 4. only
    C. 1. and 3.
    D. All of the above

595. In lung cancer in an adult, a tumor may cause hypercalcemia by
    A. direct invasion of bone, releasing calcium by destruction of bone mass
    B. producing a PTH or PTH-like substance
    C. both A. and B.
    D. none of the above

596. The clinician must be particularly alert for incidence of iatrogenic pneumothorax occurring in a patient who
    A. is being maintained by PEEP
    B. has Gram-negative bacterial pneumonia
    C. has pneumocystis pneumonia
    D. all of the above

597. In cor pulmonale, which of the following denotes its presence?
1. Right ventricular enlargement
2. Left ventricular enlargement
3. Right ventricular function is normal
4. Left ventricular function is normal
    A. 1. and 4.
    B. 2. and 3.
    C. 1. only
    D. 2. only

598. In diagnosing cor pulmonale or right ventricular hypertrophy, the electrocardiogram should give significant clues. Which of the following may be present?
  1. P-wave enlarged
  2. P-wave absent
  3. T-wave absent
  4. Peaked T-wave
  5. Partial or complete right bundle branch block
     A. 2., 3., and 5.
     B. 1., 3., 5., and 6.
     C. 2., 4., and 6.
     D. 1. and 3.

599. The Swan–Ganz catheter is an invaluable aid in
  A. managing the combined problem of pulmonary and left ventricular failure
  B. thermodilution determinations of cardiac output
  C. following effects of PEEP
  D. estimating tissue oxygenation by means of mixed venous oxygen tension

600. Which of the following is true of the Swan–Ganz?
  1. Measures right atrial pressure
  2. Measures pulmonary artery pressure
  3. Measures pulmonary artery wedge pressure
  4. Measures left atrial pressure
  5. Measures left ventricular pressure
  6. Measures right ventricular pressure
     A. 1., 2., and 3.
     B. 1., 2., 3., and 4.
     C. All but 6.
     D. All of the above

Explanatory Answers

520. C. Although incidence of influenza is highest in children age 5 to 9 and adults age 25 to 35, mortality is greater in infancy and those over the age of 50. In addition, pregnant women are also at increased risk of death from influenza. (**Ref.** 44, p. 12)

521. B. Influenza is best controlled by vaccination for persons at increased risk of fatality. They should be given annual booster shots. These include people with chronic respiratory or cardiac disease, and diabetes. (**Ref.** 44, p. 13)

522. C. Organisms frequently isolated from the sputum of patients with chronic bronchitis include *Klebsiella*, *staphylococci*, *streptococci*, and *pneumococci*. In the same patient, each may be more predominant from time to time. (**Ref.** 44, p. 16)

523. A. Chronic bronchitis is diagnosed as a persistant cough which produces >1 oz (30 mL) of sputum per day. It may vary in character, but is principally more predominant in the morning and evening. It is also worse in cold, damp weather than in dry, hot weather. (**Ref.** 44, p. 17)

524. B. Although there is no single specific cause of bronchiectasis, it most commonly is caused by some form of bronchial obstruction, whether by a disease process or by a foreign body. This obstruction is then accompanied by other processes, including cystic fibrosis, pneumonia, bronchitis, or tuberculosis. (**Ref.** 44, p. 20)

525. D. X-rays of patients with bronchiectasis may demonstrate three forms. These include cylindrical, saccular, and fusiform. Cylindrical bronchiectasis generally is not as serious and is of doubtful significance. (**Ref.** 44, p. 19)

526. C. Of bacterial pneumonia, *pneumococcus*, *streptococcus Klebsiella*, and *staphylococcus*, the one carrying the highest mortality is *Klebsiella*. Although rare, it is vital to isolate this organism early in the treatment of pneumococcal pneumonia. (**Ref.** 44, p. 26)

527. C. *Klebsiella* sputum itself is a cherry red color; however, when mixed, the patient may cough a rust-colored type of sputum. (**Ref.** 44, p. 28)

528. A. Chest x-rays are the best source for monitoring a patient's course with bacterial pneumonia. Although initially it may appear normal or near normal, the x-ray itself may give a clue to the causitive agent. (**Ref.** 44, p. 29)

529. A. Symptoms of bronchiectasis, which include persistant coughing and recurrent bouts of illness, prevent patients from leading normal lives. Treatment should include patient education on self-care in an effort to limit future problems. (**Ref.** 44, p. 24)

530. B. *Mycobacterium tuberculosis* is the organism which most often results in human infection and pulmonary tuberculosis. *M. bovis* is the tubercle of cattle and *M. avis* is the tubercle of birds. *M. fortuitum* is an atypical mycobacteria, producing disease that is indistinguishable from pulmonary tuberculosis. (**Ref.** 44, p. 36)

531. C. Pulmonary tuberculosis usually originates from the upper part of the lungs, as a small patch below the apex and most often on the right. (**Ref.** 44, p. 38)

532. D. Tuberculosis may be spread in the lung by direct extension in the involved lobe or into the pleural space, by way of the lymphatics to other parts of the body, or by the bloodstream should a caseous focus erode into a vein. It may go through such natural passages as the bronchi, trachea, throat, and eustachian tubes. (**Ref.** 44, p. 38)

533. D. Tuberculous pneumonia results in extensive death of lung tissue and profound toxemia (blood poisoning). (**Ref.** 44, p. 40)

534. B. Pulmonary tuberculosis is becoming an uncommon disease of the young and minor cause of death among White women. Hispanic and Black women, however, still have considerable tuberculosis and at an early age. Men, both Black and White, between 45 and 69 years of age, for unknown reasons, are the chief victims of tuberculosis. (**Ref.** 44, p. 42)

535. C. The most accurate form of discovering pulmonary tuberculosis is chest x-ray. (**Ref.** 44, p. 43)

536. B. The Mantoux test with PPD is the standard with which all other methods must be compared. The jet gun and multiple-puncture transcutaneous tests, such as the Heaf, Tine, and Mono-Vacc tests, are useful in the physician's office or in group screening. (**Ref.** 44, p. 43)

537. A. Histoplasmosis has two phases: a mycelial phase with a branching, threadlike form growing in the soil and bearing spores, and a single-cell yeastlike form growing within the body to produce disease. People inhaling the spores in dust develop a disease in which the yeast phase of the fungus multiplies by simple division within the body's cells. (**Ref.** 44, p. 50)

538. A. Those with generalized histoplasmosis form have sustained fever, rapid loss of weight, anemia, and enlargement of the liver and spleen. (**Ref.** 44, p. 52)

539. D. Complete control of tuberculosis can be accelerated by the use of isonazid for the treatment of infection, as a means of preventing disease. (**Ref.** 44, p. 46)

540. A. Histoplasmosis and coccidiodommycosis are diseases in humans produced by inhalation of dust contaminated with spores. (**Ref.** 44, pp. 50, 54)

541. B. Auscultation of asthmatics ranges from coarse wheezes to a high-pitched piping over both lungs, like the noises of a symphony orchestra tuning up or of a bagpipe band. (**Ref.** 44, p. 66)

542. D. The introduction of exact methods of measuring lung ventilation, volumes, and gas exchanges has made it possible to determine degrees of functional impairment due to emphysema. (**Ref.** 44, p. 69)

543. C. Localized emphysema produced by any condition causing scarring in the lung is called paracicatarical emphysema. (**Ref.** 44, p. 69)

544. D. More than 90% of emphysematous patients in some studies are heavy smokers—that is, smoke more than 20 cigarettes a day—indicating that such smoking is a causative factor in emphysema. (**Ref.** 44, p. 72)

545. B. The red blood count increases to compensate for lowered oxygen saturation, just as it does at high altitude. Therefore, polycythemia (a condition in which there is an excess of red corpuscles) may develop in well-established emphysema. (**Ref.** 44, p. 74)

546. D. In the final stage, the overloaded heart reaches its limit of muscular compensation and begins to fail (cor pulmonale). The destruction of a large part of the capillaries in the lungs, the effect of lowered blood oxygen in raising the pulmonary artery pressure, and the shunting of unaerated blood all play a part in overworking the right ventricle of the heart. (**Ref.** 44, pp. 72, 73)

547. D. A battery of physiological tests and formulas has been developed to diagnose emphysema. These measurements are most useful in establishing the stages of the disease from the earliest impairment of ventilation through oxygen lack and carbon dioxide accumulation to heart failure. A decreased ability to empty the lungs rapidly as shown by forced expiratory volume in 1 sec (FEV_1) and poor diffusion of gases in the lungs are basic abnormalities. It is important to know the oxygen and carbon dioxide content, and the pH of the arterial blood. (**Ref.** 44, p. 75)

548. D. Obstruction to the smaller air passages must be relieved by: (A) treating the infection; (B) thinning the secretions by an increase of fluid intake, expectorants, and humidifying or wetting agents; and (C) giving drugs that will dilate the bronchi. (**Ref.** 44, p. 75)

549. C. The bronchogenic carcinoma which occurs most frequently is squamous cell carcinoma. (**Ref.** 44, p. 77)

550. A. Typically, in early bronchogenic carcinoma, a "coin-shaped lesion" in the periphery of the lung will present on chest x-ray. It may be associated with lobar collapse or pneumonia. Asthma and emphysema are manifested by hyperaeration while tuberculosis is manifested by patchy infiltrations with cavity formations followed later by scarring. (**Ref.** 44, p. 83)

551. D. For inpatients who are able to maintain effective alveolar ventilation but remain hypoxemic secondary to V/Q abnormalities or intrapulmonary shunting, CPAP is the treatment of choice. Controlled or assisted ventilation is implemented for patients who cannot effectively eliminate CO_2. (**Ref.** 45, p. 84)

552. B. In cases of ARDS (Adult Respiratory Distress Syndrome), high peak airway pressures and large tidal volumes are required to effectively ventilate patients due to their decreased compliance. Low pressures and low tidal volumes may result in CO_2 retention. (**Ref.** 45, p. 84)

553. D. High-Frequency Ventilation has been useful with several scenarios. These include bronchopleural fistula. Due to the low delivered tidal volumes, less ventilation is lost through the fistula. Because of the effective alveolar ventilation at low airway pressures, it is also employed for refractory cases of hyaline membrane disease and diaphragmatic hernias (**Ref.** 45, p. 84)

554. A. Complications associated with mechanical ventilation include decreased cardiac output secondary to decreased venous return to the right ventricle, altered cerebral blood flow or increased intracranial pressure secondary to decreased venous return from the superior vena cava, and V/Q abnormalities due to ventilation on unperfused areas of lung. (**Ref.** 45, p. 86)

555. D. With mechanical ventilation, increased airway pressures may result in pneumothorax also causing subcutaneous emphysema. Vascular air embolization and pneumomediastinum may also result from positive pressure. (**Ref.** 45, p. 86)

556. C. In severe cases of respiratory distress, oxygen consumption may account for as much as 30% of total body oxygen consumption. This is especially important when oxygen availability is reduced in certain disease states. (**Ref.** 45, p. 86)

557. C. Once artificial ventilation is instituted, specific parameters must be implemented, including tidal volume (10 to 15 mL/kg), respiratory rate (generally 8 to 12 breaths/min, and flow rates adequate to meet or exceed a patient's spontaneous flow rate. I : E ratios normally are 1 : 2, but in cases of airway obstruction may be as high as 1 : 4. FIO_2 is dependent upon PAO_2 and PEEP is dependent upon the degree of refractory hypoxemia. (**Ref.** 46, p. 28)

558. B. Ventilatory rates in the range of 8 to 12 breaths/min usually are sufficient to maintain adequate alveolar ventilation. This is dependent upon the adequacy of perfusion and other physiologic parameters. (**Ref.** 46, p. 29)

559. C. Patients with obstructive airway disease may need I : E ratios of 1 : 4 to provide adequate time for exhalation. (**Ref.** 46, p. 29)

560. B. When ventilating small children, it is especially important to pay attention to compressible volume. Depending upon the patient's compliance and the type of tubing used, up to 50% of the set tidal volume may be lost to compression. (**Ref.** 46, p. 29)

561. A. During mechanical ventilation it is common to use tidal volumes that approximate 10 to 15 mL/kg. Although this is larger than the volume typically inspired in spontaneous breaths, it has been shown that volumes lower than this often lead to atelectasis. (**Ref.** 46, p. 29)

562. D. Flow rates should be set to provide for patient comfort, low airway turbulance, and sufficient time for pulmonary emptying. Generally, flow rates which supply an inspiratory time of 1 to 1½ sec are adequate. (**Ref.** 46, p. 29)

563. D. When mechanical ventilation is required following laryngoscopy, bronchoscopy, thoractomy, and neurosurgery, High-Frequency Ventilation may be instituted secondary to its low airway pressures, thereby decreasing the incidence of pulmonary trauma. (**Ref.** 46, p. 30)

564. D. A few of many causes of respiratory failure may include hemorrhagic pancreatitis, inspiration of gastric contents, and fat emboli. These problems can lead to what is known as ARDS. (**Ref.** 47, p. 3)

565. D. Central venous pressure is the best indication of intravascular volume status. In addition it reflects any compromise of right ventricular function. Normal pressures range from −1 to 7 mmHg.

566. A. Left ventricular function can be assessed either through a pulmonary artery wedge pressure (normal 6 to 12 mmHg) or by the pulmonary artery diastolic pressure in the absence of mitral stenosis or mitral regurgitation. (**Ref.** 47, p. 6)

567. D. Any injury compromising the ability to perform endotracheal intubation should be treated with an emergency tracheostomy. These include severe facial fractures, massive intraoral bleeding, laryngotracheal injury, or cervical spine injury. (**Ref.** 49, p. 12)

568. A. When a single rib is fractured in two places it is considered a flail segment. Care should be taken with patients having this type of fracture, and treatment may include mechanical ventilation for internal stabilization or surgical stabilization. (**Ref.** 49, p. 19)

569. D. Increases in the partial pressure of expired CO_2 may be caused by hypoventilation resulting in a buildup of arterial CO_2, an increase in cardiac output resulting in more CO_2 uptake from the cellular level, hyperthermia resulting in an increased CO_2 production, and rebreathing resulting in an increased deadspace ventilation. (**Ref.** 51, p. 138)

570. C. Decreases in the partial pressure of $PeCO_2$ may include hyperventilation resulting in a decreased $PaCO_2$, apnea resulting in the lack of CO_2 being expired, and reduced cardiac output which results in less blood flow into the pulmonary circulative. (**Ref.** 51, p. 138)

571. B. Negative pressure within the thoracic cavity results in an increased work of breathing and increased venous return, which may increase cardiac output. (**Ref.** 43, p. 149)

572. C. Patients with a forced vital capacity less than 70% of predicted or a forced expiratory volume of 1 sec/FVC less than 65% may be of an increased risk of postoperative pulmonary complications. For this reason, preoperative pulmonary function testing may be beneficial to predict those patients at risk. (**Ref.** 43, p. 149)

573. A. Oxygen toxicity is likely to occur at prolonged exposure to 100% oxygen at atmospheric pressure. This will result in the release of free oxygen radicals which will attack alveolar I and II type cells. FIO_2 less than 50% even at prolonged exposure is unlikely to result in oxygen toxicity. (**Ref.** 43, p. 150)

574. B. 50% of all AIDS patients have pulmonary involvement, primarily that of *Pneumocystis carnii*. (**Ref.** 58, p. 128)

575. A. Karposi's sarcoma, a vascular neoplasm, is a noninfectious complication of AIDS. Generally first noted to involve the skin, it almost always occurs in the setting of diffuse disease within the endobronchial tree. This can be confirmed by fiberoptic bronchoscopy or open lung biopsy. (**Ref.** 58, p. 130)

576. D. When obtaining mixed venous saturation blood work, samples should be drawn from the proximal port of the pulmonary arterial catheter. Aspiration should be done slowly to prevent oxygenated blood from mixing with the desired venous sample. (**Ref.** 62, p. 285)

577. E. When evaluating pulmonary artery diastolic pressures, they can be said to approximate pulmonary wedge pressures in the absence of mitral disease, pulmonary emboli, and tachycardia. Each of the situations will cause the difference between the pressures to widen. Generally the pulmonary diastolic will be higher than actual wedge pressure. (**Ref.** 62, p. 264)

578. C. To establish the diagnosis of pulmonary Karposi's sarcoma, open lung biopsy is necessary with careful selection of a grossly involved section of the lung. Therapy is limited to radiation or chemotherapy. (**Ref.** 58, p. 130)

579. B. Fractures of long bones, ribs, and the pelvis are commonly responsible for fat embolism syndrome. It is classically manifested by petechial hemorrhage. Incidence is usually exhibited 2–3 days past trauma. Early chest x-rays may be normal, but later ones exhibit fluffy infiltrates. (**Ref.** 59, p. 158)

580. D. Situations which preclude the inability to effectively cough include a central nervous system depression, displacement of the endotracheal tube, and disease conditions in which the patient becomes weak and debilitated. (**Ref.** 60, p. 196)

581. D. Infection depends upon the virulence of the invading organism and the integrity of the patient's pulmonary defense mechanisms. Chronic debilitation and malnourishment, presence of underlying chronic pulmonary disease, extensive tissue damage or resection, increased use of immunosuppressive agents in cancer therapy and transplantation surgery, and prophylactic antibiotics all increase the risk of infection following colonization. (**Ref.** 36, p. 83)

582. A. Gram-negative microbes which colonize the lower respiratory tract usually can be identified within 72 hr after intubation of the trachea. (**Ref.** 36, p. 83)

583. C. In hypoventilation oxygen therapy is of little benefit unless ventilation is restored to physiological levels. Oxygen therapy will not substitute for inadequate breathing frequency and/or tidal volume. In right-to-left shunts, oxygen therapy is of little value because of the mixing of oxygenated blood with unoxygenated blood. (**Ref.** 28, p. 269)

584. D. Indications of use of artificial airways include the following: (A) To prevent or relieve upper airway obstruction; (B) to protect the airway from aspiration; (C) to facilitate tracheal suction; and (D) to provide a sealed, closed system for mechanical ventilation or CPAP. (**Ref.** 22, p. 381)

585. D. Adverse reactions that can occur with the administration of virazole (ribavirin) include worsening of respiratory status, pneumothorax, apnea, ventilator dependence, and hypotension. **(Ref. 18)**

586. D. Factors leading to pulmonary embolism can include advanced age, bed rest, obesity, cardiac arrhythmias, and smoking. **(Ref. 61, p. 341)**

587. A. The most common symptom of pulmonary embolic disease is dyspnea. **(Ref. 61, p. 350)**

588. B. The most common physical finding of pulmonary embolic disease is tachypnea. **(Ref. 61, p. 350)**

589. B. Most patients with pulmonary embolic disease will have arterial blood gases which present acute respiratory alkalosis and hypoxemia. **(Ref. 61, p. 352)**

590. C. Alpha-antitrypsin, a serum protein that inhibits proteolytic enzymes and is under genetic control, can lead to COPD. **(Ref. 61, p. 203)**

591. B. The normal serum alpha-antitrypsin is 180 to 244 mg/dL measured by the radioimmunodiffusion technique. **(Ref. 61, p. 212)**

592. D. The most sensitive indicator of COPD that becomes abnormal first in pulmonary function is FEF 25% to 75%. **(Ref. 61, p. 211)**

593. C. The FEVC tends to remain normal until the disease is moderately advanced because COPD hinders rapid exhalation. Abnormalities are first detected in test measuring airflow rather than in the FEVC, which measures volume. **(Ref. 61, p. 211)**

594. C. The RV is increased in COPD as the airway narrows or closes during expiration because of intrinsic bronchial disease or loss of radial traction support due to emphysema. The TLC (total lung capacity) is the sum of VC + RV, and in COPD is increased by increases of RV. **(Ref. 61, p. 211)**

595. C. A tumor may cause hypercalcemia by direct invasion of bone, releasing calcium by destruction of bone mass; but another possibility is that the tumor is producing a PTH or PTH-like substance. (**Ref.** 61, p. 271)

596. D. The incidence of iatrogenic pneumothorax is a serious complication of the use of ventilators. The clinician must be particularly alert for its occurrence in patients who are being maintained by positive end-expiratory pressure (PEEP) or who have Gram-negative bacterial or pneumocystis pneumonia. (**Ref.** 61, p. 303)

597. A. Cor pulmonale denotes right ventricular enlargement secondary to an intrinsic lung disorder or inadequacy of respiratory function. Cardiac enlargement should be limited to the right ventricle, which may demonstrate dilation or hypertrophy, and left ventricular function should be normal. (**Ref.** 61, p. 369)

598. B. The electrocardiogram should give significant clue to the diagnosis of cor pulmonale. The P-waves may be enlarged, particularly in leads II, III, and AVF. Primary T-wave inversion is commonly seen. There may also be a partial or complete right bundle-branch block. (**Ref.** 61, p. 369)

599. A. The Swan–Ganz catheter has proved invaluable in managing the complex problem of combined pulmonary and left ventricular failure. (**Ref.** 61, p. 231)

600. B. The Swan–Ganz catheter allows one to measure right atrial pulmonary artery and pulmonary artery wedge (left atrial) pressures. In addition, these catheters provide capability for performing thermodilution determinations of cardiac output. (**Ref.** 61, p. 231)

References

1. Rosendorff C: *Clinical cardiovascular and pulmonary physiology*, Raven Press, New York, NY, 1983.

2. *Taber's cyclopedic medical dictionary*, Edition 12, F.A. Davis Co., Philadelphia, PA, 1974.

3. Jacob and Francone: *Structure and function in man*, 3rd Edition, W. B. Saunders Co., Philadelphia, PA, 1974.

4. Grenard, Bach, and Rich: *Introduction to respiratory therapy*, 2nd Edition, Glenn Educational Medical Service, Inc. Monsey, New York, 1971.

5. Shapiro, Harrison, and Trout: *Clinical application of respiratory care*, Year Book Medical Publishers, Inc. Chicago, Ill., 1975.

6. Wade JF: *Comprehensive respiratory care*, 3rd Edition, C.V. Mosby Co., St. Louis, MO, 1982.

7. Egan DF: *Fundamentals of respiratory therapy*, 2nd Edition, C.V. Mosby Co., St. Louis, MO, 1973.

8. Gaskell DV and Weber BA: *The Brompton Hospital guide to chest physiotherapy*, 2nd Edition, Blackwell Scientific Publications, Oxford, England, 1974.

9. Haas A, Pineda H, Haas F, Axen K: *Pulmonary therapy and rehabilitation*, Williams and Wilkins, Baltimore, Md., 1979.

10. Blodgett D: *Manual of pediatric respiratory care procedures*, J.B. Lippincott, Co., Philadelphia, PA, 1982.

11. Thacker W: *Postural drainage and respiratory control*, 2nd Edition, Lloyd-Luke Ltd., London, England, 1963.

12. Rattenborg CC and Holaday DA: Lung physiotherapy as an adjunct to surgical care, *Surg Clin No Amc* 44:219, 1964 (FEB).

13. Gray H, Edited by Gross CM: *Gray's anatomy*, 28th Edition, Lea Febiger, Philadelphia, PA, 1970.

14. Rau Jr JL: *Respiratory therapy pharmacology*, 2nd Edition, Year Book Medical Publishers, Inc., Chicago, Ill., 1975.

15. Bergersen BS: *Pharmacology in nursing*, C.V. Mosby Co., St. Louis, MO, 1973.

16. Ziment I: *Respiratory pharmacology and therapeutics*, W.B. Saunders Co., Philadelphia, PA, 1978.

17. Aderson E: *Workbook of solutions and dosages of drugs*, C.V. Mosby Co., St. Louis, MO, 1964.

18. Literature provided by manufacturers of this equipment or product.

19. Miller WF: Fundamental principles of aerosol therapy, *Respiratory Care* 17:295, 1972 (May–June).

20. Ziment I: Mucokinesis—The methodology of moving mucus, *Respiratory Therapy* 4:15, 1974 (March–April).

21. Heard SO: Drugs affecting respiration, *Current Reviews in Respiratory Therapy*, Lesson 14, Volume 7, 1985.

22. Kacmarek RM, Mack CW, Dimas S: *The essentials of respiratory therapy*, 2nd Edition, Year Book Publishers Inc., Chicago, Ill., 1985.

23. Shapiro BA: *Clinical application of blood gases*, Year Book Medical Publishers, Inc., Chicago, Ill., 1975.

24. Brooks SM: *Integrated basic science*, 3rd year, C.V. Mosby Co., St. Louis, MO, 1970.

25. Anthony CP and Kolthoff NF: *Textbook of anatomy and physiology*, 8th Edition, C.V. Mosby Co., St. Louis, MO, 1971.

26. Chaffee EE and Greisheimer EM: *Basic physiology and anatomy*, 3rd Edition, JB Lippincott Co., Philadelphia, PA, 1974.

27. Mondrow DN: Review of cardiovascular physiology for the respiratory therapist, *Current Reviews in Respiratory Therapy*, Lesson 2, Volume 7, 1984.

28. Eubanks DH and Bonc RC: *Comprehensive respiratory care*, C.V. Mosby Co., St. Louis, MO, 1985.

29. Gal TJ: Approach to preoperative pulmonary evaluation and preparation, *Current Reviews in Respiratory and Critical Care*, Lesson 21, Volume 9, 1987.

30. Gal TJ: Perioperative approach to patients with chronic obstructive pulmonary disease, *Current Reviews in Respiratory Therapy*, Lesson 4, Volume 8, 1985.

31. Benumof JL: Regulation of the pulmonary circulation, *Current Reviews in Respiratory Therapy*, Lesson 8, Volume 8, 1985.

32. Beachey W: Physiologic buffering systems, *Current Reviews in Respiratory Therapy*, Lesson 12, Volume 8, 1986.

33. Boysen PG: Management of perioperative respiratory dysfunction, *Current Reviews in Respiratory Therapy*, Lesson 21, Volume 8, 1986.

34. Darvich-Kodjouri C: Care of the patient with a new tracheostomy, *Current Reviews in Respiratory and Critical Care*, Lesson 6, Volume 10, 1987.

35. Bowton DL: Bronchodilator therapy, *Current Reviews in Respiratory and Critical Care*, Lesson 8, Volume 9, 1987.

36. Darin J: Respiratory therapy equipment and the development of nasocomial respiratory tract infections, *Current Reviews in Respiratory Therapy*, Lesson 11, Volume 4, 1982.

37. Bartley J: Legionella, clinical features and an epidemiological investigation, *Current Reviews in Respiratory Therapy*, Lesson 1, Volume 7, 1984.

38. Berry AJ: AIDS and hepatitis B, occupational hazards, *Current Reviews in Respiratory and Critical Care*, Lesson 11, Volume 10, 1988.

39. "Pin index safety system for flush type cylinder valves" (Pamphlet V-2), Compressed Gas Association, New York, NY

40. "Diameter index safety system" (Pamphlet V-6), Compressed Gas Association, New York, NY.

41. "Inhalation therapy" (Pamphlet 56-B), National Fire Protection Association, Boston, MA, 1968.

42. Smith RA and Kirby RR: Current concepts in respiratory care, Part I, *Current Reviews in Respiratory Therapy*, Lesson 18, Volume 8, 1986.

43. Smith RA and Kirby RR: Current concepts in respiratory care, Part II, *Current Reviews in Respiratory Therapy*, Lesson 19, Volume 8, 1986.

44. *Introduction to lung diseases*, 5th Edition, American Lung Association, 1973.

45. Kirby RR and Smith RA: Current concepts in mechanical ventilation, *Current Reviews in Respiratory Therapy*, Lesson 11, Volume 8, 1986.

46. Parker J and Raffin T: Mechanical ventilator support, current tecnhiques and recent advances, *Current Reviews in Respiratory and Critical Care*, Lesson 4, Volume 9, 1986.

47. Kirby RR: Current concepts in hemorrhagic shock, *Current Reviews in Respiratory and Critical Care*, Lesson 1, Volume 9, 1986.

48. Banner MJ: Technical aspects of high-frequency ventilation, *Current Reviews in Respiratory Therapy*, Lesson 12, Volume 7, 1985.

49. Mathisi DJ: Thoracic trauma, *Current Reviews in Respiratory and Critical Care*, Lesson 3, Volume 9, 1986.

50. Gilmartin M and Make BJ: Mechanical ventilation in the home, *Current Reviews in Respiratory Therapy*, Lesson 18, Volume 7, 1985.

51. Smith RA: Monitoring mechanical ventilators, Part I, *Current Reviews in Respiratory and Critical Care,* Lesson 17, Volume 9, 1987.

52. McLaughlin G: Respiratory gas monitoring, *Current Reviews in Respiratory Therapy*, Lesson 2, Volume 8, 1985.

53. Hill TM and Sorbello JG: "Humidity outputs of large-reservoir nebulizers," *Respiratory Care*, Volume 32, Number 4, April 1987.

54. Rau Jr JF and May, DF: "The effects of heated and unheated distilled water aerosols on expiratory flowrates in persons with normal pulmonary functions," *Respiratory Care*, Volume 32, Number 12, December 1987.

55. Orlando III R, Chinniah N, Riegle C, Morris B: High-frequency jet ventilation, *Current Reviews in Respiratory Therapy*, Lesson 9, Volume 8, 1985.

56. Capps JS, Ritz R, Pierson DJ: "An evaluation in four ventilators of characteristics that affect work of breathing," *Respiratory Care*, Volume 32, Number 11, November 1987.

57. Hess D and Gretchen G: "The effects of two-hand versus one-hand ventilation on volumes delivered during bag-ventilation at various resistances and compliances," *Respiratory Care*, Volume 32, Number 11, November 1987.

58. Villanueva AG and Farber HW: Pulmonary complications in AIDS patients, *Current Reviews in Respiratory and Critical Care*, Lesson 16, Volume 9, 1987.

59. Steingrub JR and Teres D: Pulmonary fat embolism syndrome, *Current Reviews in Respiratory Therapy*, Lesson 20, Volume 8, 1986.

60. Rarey KP and Youtsey JW: *Respiratory patient care*, NJ: Prentice-Hall, 1981.

61. Gracey DR: *Pulmonary disease in the adult*, Year Book Medical Publishers, Inc., Chicago, Ill., 1981.

62. Pierson DJ: *Respiratory intensive care*, Daedalus Enterprises Inc., 1986.